Everyday Devotion

The Heart of Being

Guru Prem Singh Khalsa

Kundalini Research Institute

Training ❀ Publishing ❀ Research ❀ Resources

© 2011 Guru Prem Singh Khalsa

Published by the Kundalini Research Institute

PO Box 1819
Santa Cruz, NM 87532
www.kundaliniresearchinstitute.org
ISBN 978-1-934532-75-1

This publication has received the KRI Seal of Approval. This Seal is given only to products that have been reviewed for accuracy and integrity of the sections containing the 3HO lifestyle and Kundalini Yoga as taught by Yogi Bhajan®.

Editor: Sat Purkh Kaur Khalsa
KRI Review: Siri Neel Kaur Khalsa
Consulting Editor: Nirvair Singh Khalsa
Copy Editor: Tara Joffe
Design and Layout: Prana Projects: Ditta Khalsa, Biljana Nedelkovska
Photography: Alan Miyatake, Toyo Miyatake Studio. Photoshoot art direction and edits by Ravitej Khalsa
Models: Guru Prem Singh Khalsa and Simran Kaur Khalsa

Devotion is a very rare process in life; if you allow it to, it will eat up your ego.
—Yogi Bhajan[1]

1   © The Teachings of Yogi Bhajan, July 28, 1982

Acknowledgements

I am deeply grateful for my journey, for my soul's longing, which brought me to the feet of the Guru and the recognition of God within and without!

I would like to share my gratitude for all who made this book possible. To every teacher, student, friend and family member, "Thank you," you have all played an important part in the mosaic that is my life.

I would like to thank Nirvair Singh for offering me the opportunity to write this book, I really appreciate his faith in allowing me to represent our community by sharing my adventures in transformation.

The telling of my story required a great effort from a few people. If I'd known I was going to become a writer, I would have studied English. Fortunately, I have an editor who did, Sat Purkh Kaur Khalsa, who has been invaluable in this process, and has made it sound as if I had indeed studied English. How many people get to write a book and receive a creative writing tutorial in the process? I did, and thank you.

A very special thank you to my wife, Simran, who allowed me the space and time to write, and for her assistance in writing this book. To her parents, Sat Jivan Singh and Sat Jivan Kaur for having her and for their invaluable input! And of course where would I be without my parents? Among the many things I am grateful for is that they chose to raise their family in West Los Angeles. Because of where I grew up, the Dharma was in my own "back yard," waiting for me to wake up!

To all of my teachers who I have been fortunate enough to learn from, and who have been a part of my growth and awakening, thank you. Any wisdom I've acquired is because of my teachers, and it's on their shoulders that I stand.

Yogi Bhajan, also known as the Siri Singh Sahib, requires special mention, it is because of his efforts and faith in me that I had a chance to change my life from living in the shadows to living in the light. By his efforts and the Guru's teachings, and all my many blessings, I have been able to live a healthy, happy and holy life.

To the rest of my teachers, many of whom I write about, a deep gratitude for all that you shared. I apologize to anyone not properly acknowledged.

And finally to my daughter and son, Hari Simran Kaur and Siri Guru Dev Singh, thank you for smiling back at me, it feels like a reflection of the success I've had as a parent, student and teacher.

Sat Nam,
Guru Prem Singh Khalsa

For decades Yogi Bhajan taught Kundalini Yoga, meditation and yogic lifestyle a couple of evenings a week, and then on Sundays, he would change his hat (figuratively), and as the Siri Singh Sahib give a lecture on Sikh Dharma.[2] These two paths overlapped in many ways, including the Shabad Guru,[3] chanting mantras, which include God's many names, and the overall idea that we are infinite beings here to have a human experience. He wanted us to awaken and recognize our true identity, Sat Nam, and live a healthy, happy and holy lifestyle, with commitment, dignity, divinity and grace. And it is to these teachings that this book is dedicated.

2 Sikh Path of Righteous
3 The Shabad Guru is the sound current of the Guru's vibration. It is the everlasting word which has the effect of infinity, so man by his nature can grow into reality, cutting through the clouds and storms to become crystal clear to see the path to his destiny.

Table of Contents

An Experience of Mastery

One evening in the late 1990s, I went to visit my spiritual teacher Yogi Bhajan, also known as the Siri Singh Sahib. As was often the case, I was called to give him a massage and other treatments. When I arrived, I noticed that there were probably 20 people in the living room with him. I greeted him in the usual respectful manner. But before I could sit down, Yogi Bhajan spoke to the whole room, deciding right then that I needed an official title. I had little notion of what to expect or of why I needed a title. It was both humbling and embarrassing to be standing in the middle of this naming process. Yogi Bhajan finally settled on a title—Posture Master. With this newly bestowed title, he asked how I felt and what I thought. I replied, "I'll try not to slouch."

Yet I didn't feel at all like a master of anything, even postures. Was this another test? Or was it a gift delivered early? I decided that it was a gift and that I could unwrap it in my own way. I didn't know of anyone else to whom Yogi Bhajan had given the title of Master. But I did recall his stories of receiving his own title, Master of Kundalini Yoga, when the title was given to him, he just accepted it and became it. I had already learned how to receive gifts from my spiritual teacher, when he gave me his poems to put to music. With that gift, I learned to listen for the melodies and arrangements that came with his poems. Now I had this title and responsibility to be the Posture Master. With this new gift, I decided I would once again listen so I could learn what to do with it.

For years I had taken advantage of any opportunity to ask Yogi Bhajan about yoga and its various protocols. Some of these talks were just between the two of us; others were with various people in the living room. I received numerous tutorials on various aspects of Kundalini Yoga. The nature of any type of true mastery requires teaching. Yogi Bhajan taught that to learn about something we should read about it. To know something well, we should write about it. And to master something, we should teach it.

Thus, part of the Posture Master package of knowing was to write books on Kundalini Yoga. I have written three so far, including this one. I also needed to expand my teaching sphere, which I've done through my involvement in worldwide Kundalini Yoga teacher training programs. But what became the most interesting part of this process was my plan to learn all 84 major asanas.[4] One reason I embarked on the adventure—what I called "The 84"—was that this is what Yogi Bhajan had done earlier in his life. But I also had deeper and more compelling reasons for this adventure. I was determined to become an expert on how to do and teach even the

4 Comfortable seat, Yogic posture

most difficult kriyas,[5] as there were numerous kriyas and asanas that I found very difficult to do or, for that matter, teach. I was 44 years old, and my second child had just been born. I felt very rusty for a Posture Master; I needed to get in shape.

What better way to get in shape than to have a goal? In order to learn the difficult kriyas and all of the postures, I began to supplement my kundalini practice with the study of other yoga styles because, as I saw it, there was no other way to get the necessary technical guidance for learning the asanas. In many ways, it was like I had returned to gymnastics training. I was breaking my body down and rebuilding it in a far subtler way and with much better alignment. I am my own favorite toy, and doing yoga asanas for me is a lot of fun.

Between 1995 and 2005 was a really wonderful period in my relationship with Yogi Bhajan. I had been through the big tests, some of which I share throughout this book and some to be saved for another time. This was also my deep yoga asana period. I was determined to become worthy of the Posture Master title, and Yogi Bhajan was in my corner. This also marked the first time in my relationship with him that I would offer disagreements on the subject of yoga, though I must say that it is very difficult to have a discussion in which you disagree with his wisdom. But all of my disagreements were about teaching protocols.

When Yogi Bhajan first began teaching in the United States, he had been very hands-on. Through the years, though, he became more and more subtle. He used the power of his voice more then the power of his hands. I came to realize that he was focusing more on dharma building than on body building. Much of the technical aspects of Kundalini Yoga, in terms of physical form and alignment, he deferred to me. This left me with countless questions, and he

5 Specific combination of yogic posture, hand position, breathing and mantra: literally a complete action.

was available to discuss them with me. He rarely gave me directives but instead brought me to clarity to understand the bigger picture and the greater importance.

What I learned most from these discussions was to listen even more deeply. A few of the subjects we discussed include the different variations of Breath of Fire, variations of Sat Kriya, *Surya Namaskar* or Sun Salutes, the Professional Anger Kriya,[6] and five different ways of doing Sarbandanday Kriyas. I was constantly asking about teaching methods—use of props? Yes, but without breaking the flow of kriya. Hands-on assistance? Not in a typical Kundalini Yoga class, but there are always therapeutic exceptions. Don't we ever do headstands? Not usually, however headstands have been taught in unique individual circumstances. During one such yoga meeting, the subject of Kundalini Yoga warm-ups was discussed. I asked whether Sun Salutations would be the appropriate way to warm up. Yogi Bhajan's response was, "We always did Surya Namaskars before kriya, when the sun would be rising at fifteen degrees." I then asked what style of Sun Salutation he recommended; he challenged me with a response of, "Figure it out!" There are at least six different ways to do these classic exercises. I wasn't sure that I knew enough to figure it out. But I decided that part of my adventure with the 84 asanas was to collect as much information as I could about the greater world of yoga so I could figure it out.

The idea of gathering the greater knowledge was part of earlier Sikh history. Guru Gobind Singh, the Tenth Sikh Guru,[7] sent a few well-chosen students to all parts of India to gather the Vedic,[8] Yogic, and artistic knowledge; compile it; and bring it back to Anandpur Sahib.[9] In a similar spirit, I studied, read countless books, and sought out the best teachers of many traditions. I visited so many outer schools

6 from *The Heart Rules* by Guru Prem Singh Khalsa
7 Guru means enlightener, literally that which takes us from darkness to light.
8 Ancient Hindu text, covering a vast body of knowledge, including Vedanta philosophy
9 A town fortress in Punjab India.

and inner places that I began to believe I was traveling through the land of Oz in search of the Wizard of Wisdom. Along the way in my outer world, I met many interesting teachers and fellow travelers. I realized that after 10 years of learning the asanas—or as I like to refer to them, "the body alphabet"—karmas of past emotions were leaving my body, while other attachments of a new sort were starting to accumulate.

Unfortunately, my ego was still very present, and I wanted more and more from these postures. I had already received what I came for, but I wanted more! So I did more, more, and more advanced asanas. I was back to conquering the postures instead of embracing their wisdom. By this time, Yogi Bhajan had passed away, and there was no physical teacher to confer with. What was supposed to be a limited journey to the land of asanas had become an extended adventure.

And then it happened. I got injured. I injured my back and couldn't do my "hobby." It took more than a year to heal, but I eventually got back on track. I rediscovered my direction when I began writing my second book, *The Heart Rules*. I was searching for feelings from my body and realized it was time to reconnect to the subtle feelings of my soul. My heart was calling: "You've been away long enough; it's time to come back." This felt like a combination of the prodigal son and Dorothy's adventure in Oz. In a way, I had spent all of that energy just so I could learn; all I needed, was to click my heels three times and say, "*Sat Nam Wahe Guru*."[10] I realized that there is no place like home. Of course, now I know that home is where the heart is, and if something is good, take it to heart.

10 Truth is my identity, Wow! Great is God!

An Invitation

It was in December 2009, while I visited my wife's family in Española, New Mexico, that I was first approached by Nirvair Singh Khalsa, president of the Kundalini Research Institute, to write a book about Kundalini Yoga and *Sikh Dharma*, the Sikh path of rightous living.

I said yes immediately, without giving it much thought. Having agreed, however, I then began to think, What did I just agree to do? It was a very big undertaking, and I began to doubt that I was really qualified to write such a book. Then when I began to listen deeply within myself, I recognized that the book they wanted was, in essence, already written inside of me. The challenge was getting it out. As it turns out, this book is really just my story of how I came to be me, Guru Prem Singh Khalsa. This tale of transformation has five purposes: to entertain, educate, exercise, elevate, and empower. So if I tell a good story that brings you new understandings, inspires you to perspire, raises your spirits, and gets you to live a life that brings you closer to your own destiny, then I will be happy with these efforts.

I grew up with secrets—secrets that, because of my upbringing, I had to keep to myself. My biggest secret was that I believed that God existed and lived within me. That doesn't sound so revolutionary today, but in the postwar boom that was Southern California, the notion of God, within you or outside of you, was not in fashion. You have to understand, my parents lived through and fought in World War II. From that point on, they were living in a kind of post-Holocaust neurosis: How could there be a God if there was so much suffering in the world, which God supposedly created from love? Humankind had become the moral authority that would protect the world from future tyranny—God was rejected, and my parents essentially became atheists. Reverence for God was considered a weakness, so my experience of a loving God who lived in and ruled my heart, head and mind had to be pushed away.

I never spoke of my deep-seated beliefs and pretended, for the benefit of my family and the world, that I too was a nonbeliever. In my efforts to fit into my family and the world, I slowly turned away from my own inner knowing and was left with a profound and painful emptiness, which could only be abated by outside attention. I substituted piety for precision, and in a relatively short amount of time, I became accomplished in both sports and music.

I chased the world and ran from God. This was my deal with the Devil: I'd be rewarded now but would have to pay later. With this bargain in place, I could do bad in order to feel good and defer the consequences. Yet underneath it all, I always believed that God was waiting for me. I lived with this secret for many years. Meanwhile, I envied my openly religious friends and longed to be part of a congregation of devotees who openly worshipped the One God.

The only thing that placated my pain was drawing attention to myself from the outside world. I willingly traded my character and my values for short-term benefits. I did what I wanted to feel good. Luckily for me, those things weren't too bad—that is, they weren't terribly immoral or illegal. Instead, I became very disciplined and skilled in ways that would provide me with a steady supply of attention—ego-feeding attention. I craved attention and developed devices to get it. But being good at my chosen endeavors was often not enough. I would also lie about and embellish my talents. In my mind, I was only guilty if I got caught.

I was buying time because I didn't know how to pass time. My loneliness grew deeper as my soul grew darker. I couldn't validate myself, so I began to depend more and more upon the outside world to validate me. I learned early how to press people for attention, appreciation, and admiration. I impressed them with the Devil's own device—the ability to amaze people. Amazement gains you entry into another person's psyche.

I learned the art of amazement by being amazed myself. When I was about seven years old, I watched gymnasts practice at the recreation center next door. I believed that if I could do those tricks, then I could impress and amaze people, too. So I signed myself up, thus beginning an adventure that would help define my identity for the next 15 years. I became highly skilled at gymnastics and was somewhat well-known for my competitive success. I had the ability to do what seemed impossible with my flips and twists. It was so powerful; with this skill, I could instantly make myself the center of attention. I approached music with the same purpose—to impress—whether on the piano, drums, or guitar. My interest wasn't in the music or its beauty alone, instead it was a means to an end—your energy beaming at me!

My only motivation for working hard in school was so that I could one day attend a prestigious university. I had a strong body but a weak spirit, and all my efforts served to grow my ego but not my true Self. I was trying to fill the hole in my heart, and, like all compulsives, enough was never enough. Ultimately my experiences in college brought me to such a dark state that the flicker of my soul's light could finally be seen. This was the first act of grace: somehow, through my own cleverness and deception, I ended up in a Kundalini Yoga class. I wanted to meet this girl who I had been watching from a distance. I learned she was a vegetarian who didn't care for meat eaters. I decided to become a vegetarian just so she would talk to me. The day I finally introduced myself, I had been a vegetarian for about four hours! That and the fact that I brought my parents new puppy to class was enough for her to invite me to her yoga and mime class—and that was my beginning.

The teacher, whose name was Charlie, was one of Yogi Bhajan's first students in Los Angeles. I didn't know it at the time, but Charlie was dying of cancer. His enthusiasm never revealed his illness. He taught Kundalini Yoga as a part of his mime class. Kundalini Yoga prepared students for the subtle skill that a mime would need. At that time, I was anything but subtle. I was living in a body-mind filled with excessive tension. I was controlled but not calm. Charlie saw through my act and began to help me become free from the misguided limitations of my body, mind, and ego. It was there that I began to become aware of my emotional confinement. My gymnastic strength had kept me from experiencing the deeper tension that lay beneath the surface. By my third class, I was beginning to awaken from my dark sleep. I realized that much of my life had been motivated by fear and anger, and the yoga was beginning to help me recognize it. I soon realized that this was my chance at a new life, one in which the possibility of happiness was obtainable.

After about four or five kundalini and mime classes, Charlie suggested that I take a class at Guru Ram Das Ashram. Upon arriving at the ashram, I recognized the place as a Sikh temple. By then, I was already a bit familiar with the Kundalini Yoga Sikh community because a close friend from high school had been one of the first students of Yogi Bhajan's to convert to the Sikh lifestyle. Four years later, I found myself in the Guru Ram Das Ashram curious and receptive. This was the second moment of grace.

When I first sat down in the ashram, I felt that I was sitting in a sacred place. The reverence people showed to the building and its artifacts was special. During my first Kundalini Yoga class in the ashram, I was seated toward the back. There was a curtained area behind me, and somebody was singing in a soft voice that sounded like a cross between a confessional and a divine hymn. What I didn't know at the time was that the ashram was both a yoga center and a *gurdwara* (a Sikh house of worship). What I was hearing was what is known as an Akhand Path (a continuous reading of the Sikh scriptures). I was struck by the sound of the person behind the curtain. Although the words were spoken quietly, they drew me in. After class, I asked the teacher what was happening behind the curtain. She explained that there was a continuous reading of the *Siri Guru Granth Sahib*,[11] which is the Guru brought to light and life through the sound current and the praising of the name of God.

11 The living Guru of the Sikhs

This was my introduction to the *bhakti*[12] path within Kundalini Yoga. I soon learned that the *shakti*[13] energy that Kundalini Yoga awakened was incomplete without *bhakti*, or devotion.

But what was I to be devoted to? I learned that we become devoted to our own inner virtue, because without inner virtue there can be no true devotion. Thus began my journey to recognize and refine my inner virtue. With this Guru as my guide, my journey to self-realization and fulfillment began.

Becoming Human

We all want to feel good, right? And if we don't quite know what "good" feels like, then we know that we at least want to feel better. The problem is that there are countless ways to feel good without being a human being. We do good or bad things to feel differently. And that's the starting point for many of us. But what we want is to be good. Being good is when our good will is God's will—to be able to transcend the ego and witness the virtues acting within us, becoming us. To succeed, it is important to explain the goal of being human. Yogi Bhajan defined being human like this: *Hu* means "spectrum of light," as in the hues of light refracting from a prism. The colors seen and unseen become the various colors that emanate from the pure white light. The light spectrum radiating from the pure light of the soul is the *Hu*. *Man* is defined as "mind." So, what do we mean when we say *human being*? In this case, we mean dwelling at ease in the illuminated mind—becoming a being of light.

Our desire to "be good" gives birth to virtues and morals. *Virtue* is often defined as moral excellence; so, to be virtuous is to excel at morality. But why are we, as humans, so concerned with virtues and morals anyway? Because, as humans, we are self-conscious;

12 Yogic path of devotion
13 Feminine aspect of God, God's power manifested.

and therefore, we live with the consequences of our decisions. Likewise, because we must live in the consequences, we are, by design, created to live by a comparative, comprehensive, and intuitive mind. As a kid, I had the comparative mind down. I saw what others got, and I saw how I could get it. But as I matured, I recognized that getting what I wanted—especially getting it through my ego—wasn't, and never would be, enough. I needed to find a way back to my True Heart. I needed to cultivate my sense of the whole-hearted life, the good life; I needed to connect to my intuition. That's when I met my spiritual teacher who showed me that the virtues of life, the disciplines of the good life, could fulfill me more than any of the things I had been grasping for. I could quit trying to impress others and begin cultivating my capacity to affect others for the good. The path of virtue leads from the True Heart to the Pure Heart. But in my journey, I had to learn that doing good is not the same as being good.

If ego is the disease, it may also have within it the seeds of a cure. When the ego is used to satisfy temporary emotions and feelings, it compromises our character and leads us away from virtue—even when we're doing good. In the beginning, we often do good to feel good. But just as often, we might do bad to feel good. Our egos like to impress people with our talent, skills, power, beauty—you name it, we'll use it to impress. But doing good to impress or gain attention often comes with some painful karmas: "No good deed goes unpunished."

Spiritual maturity requires that we discern the difference between impacting and impressing. The karmic law of *ahimsa* means "to do no harm." When we aim to impress others by how kind we are, how generous we are, how helpful we are, we perpetrate a subtle form of violence because it is a manipulation. When we try to impress, we act from selfish motives, and our contribution is conditional. But when we allow our virtues to impact, we are not seeking to gain from our actions, especially at the expense of others. Our kindness, courage, and generosity achieve their fullest impact because they are done without false motives; we've dropped ego gratification and moved toward true virtue.

In the process of becoming good, however, our ego-based actions are rewarded with feeling better. It feels good to act kindly, to stand up for righteousness, to practice good manners. But when our consciousness is not developed enough, we often do things to feel good, such as abuse drinking, smoking, drugs, food or sex to achieve that same good feeling. What we can do to feel good is endless, and our ego will do anything—good or bad—to feel better. If our identity isn't fed from an authenticity of the heart, from a union with God, from a deep, internal fulfillment, then we sometimes act out destructively to fill up that void. The cultivation of the intuitive mind allows our creativity to manifest within that same void—our relationship to it now is *shuniya*, a conscious state of zero, an experience of oneness, being fully present rather than a feeling of isolation and loneliness. We are able to act without ego, and therefore our actions become creative, intuitive, productive— loving—rather than destructive.

Although the path of higher consciousness often begins by doing good for a reward, we have to move beyond this reward-based behavior in order to experience our true virtues. Doing good for a reward is modeled for us from an early age. Parents practice this with their children: Do your homework and then you may watch TV. With food, it has been institutionalized, with dessert coming at the end of the meal. Even with exercise: "If I work out for two hours then I can eat whatever I want," or "If I train for a marathon,

I will have the body I always wanted." This ego-grasping behavior never allows us to experience the gift of receiving. We constantly strive for that next thing that will deliver us to the feeling we want to have. This pattern sets us up for a constant state of hunger— never being truly fulfilled but only filled up. We also can fall into the trap of chasing bigger lives, but not necessarily better ones. To truly be human we have to live our virtues out of our own natural expression of joy, delight, and service, not because we're hoping for some feeling or some experience.

In fact, the goal of the virtuous life is to become a Human Being— that is, a spiritual being having a human experience. But, how can simply living a human life be virtuous? How can simply becoming a human being be the end game? Cultivating the virtues means that we cultivate the qualities of the divine aspects of God within us. So, just as we live the virtues of life, we become the divine here on Earth. The English language makes it easier to understand virtue because it is described as heart metaphors. The virtues are known by the hearts they represent: warm-hearted, true-hearted, brave-hearted, whole-hearted. These terms are generally not used to describe a single, individual act, but instead an entire moral character or quality.

The heart is also described as the mind. In the Old Testament, *heart* is used throughout as a reference to the mind. When Tibetans say "mind," they touch their heart center. So, if *human* means the full-spectrum mind, or the enlightened mind, then what is this mind? Let's talk about how it is, rather than what it is for now. Our bodies, with their trillions of cells, organize the brain, which itself is part of those same trillions of cells, giving the mind its interactions with the world. Our actions and reactions are constantly programming and reprogramming our brains, and our minds reflect this.

The virtues create a light in the human heart, and this light contributes to what is known as the Radiant Body. This radiance culminates in our individual majesty, our royal qualities. It is the culmination of the practice of Raj Yoga, the practice of becoming majestic, noble, royal and humble wherein the soul, within the Heart of Virtues rules the mind and body. *Being* means "in the present" or "in the immortal Now." The fundamental problem lies in the mind; the mind, unless trained, does not know how to be in the present. Because it is so difficult being in the present, and yet so painful not being in the present, we do what we do to feel better. Yet when we live only for temporary emotional satisfaction, shadows are cast upon the heart. These shadows are also described in "heart" language: cold-hearted, stone-hearted, broken-hearted, cheatin'-hearted. Our actions often distance us from the light of the True Heart. But the Pure Heart is only bestowed—a gift of grace from the true Guru.

We cannot make ourselves pure. In fact the very path to the pure heart leaves some impurities from the challenges faced and overcome. We cannot, by our own virtuous ego, become pure hearted; for even a virtuous ego leaves behind residues and impurities, which can make us stronger—but not pure. We can prepare to be purified and this preparation is the journey of Dharma, or path of righteousness. On this path we develop our heart. We use our gifts and talents to achieve virtue. And we cultivate our intuition, compassion, and creativity to become fully human. The practice of Raj Yog is the path to becoming a human being. The True Heart is where the journey of Raj Yoga begins. Our foundation is Kundalini Yoga as taught by Yogi Bhajan.® And so our journey begins.

Chapter One

Journey to the Heart

Most of us, at one point or another, must make this journey—from our heads to our hearts, from our ego to our soul, from thinking to deep listening, from outside to inside. This is the story of my own journey.

My younger life was defined by my discipline, but I used it to chase my own ego. When I retired from gymnastic competition at age 23, my greatest fear was not having a discipline with which to define myself. Thus began my search for new disciplines. Yoga and martial arts quickly replaced my gymnastics. But my old motivations were still in place. In the early days of my Kundalini Yoga practice, I studied other spiritual practices. I was introduced to Taoism through the study and practice of Tai Chi, Kung Fu, and Taoist healing arts. I was very blessed to be studying with two masters at the time, Yogi Bhajan and Master Ni.

Master Ni taught me a great deal about mindfulness in everyday life. In my study with him, I prided myself on my discipline and hard work. One day Master Ni came up to me and asked, "Working hard?" To which I replied, "Yes, Sir, I am working very hard." He nodded his head and walked on. About a week later, he asked me the same question, "Working hard?" Again, I replied, "Yes, Sir, I am working very hard." A few weeks after that, Master Ni approached me again, but this time in a very stern manner and asked, "Are you still working hard?" Well, now I was confused. So I replied, "I think I'm working hard." With that, Master Ni began to laugh and walked away. After about six steps, he turned around and said, "I never work hard; I just work." His words have stuck with me ever since. Master Ni was a master at using the correct amount of chi for whatever task he was doing. I, on the other hand, worked hard to make a favorable impression. Yet working hard for the wrong reasons denies the gifts that only devoted service can bring. Thus began an awakening of consciousness: I was here to impact, not impress, and in order to be effective, the work I did for myself and the world had to be selfless. This was not a lesson I learned quickly.

The need to impress was a survival mechanism that I had been using since I was five years old. That mechanism represented the constant struggle between my temporary emotional satisfaction and experiencing the healing nectar of God's love. But at the time of my early yogic development, during my search for a new discipline to define my life, I knew that I could move no further by serving solely my ego. Instead, my ego needed to be trained to serve my soul. A choice had to be made; but which path would I choose?

I had studied other religions. Having been born into a culturally Jewish but secular family, I thought that I should begin with Judaism. I had a family friend who was a rabbi. Rabbi Bob, as he was known, had been part of my family for about 11 years. Although it was surprising that my parents would be in the regular company of a rabbi, I understood that he served as my family's moral compass. Yet for myself, morality was irrelevant without a God or supreme reality. I believed morality could easily be compromised without some constant to depend upon; I didn't want to sign up for moral relativism. I needed to know what lay hidden behind the curtain of my own consciousness.

Through numerous conversations with Rabbi Bob, I explored how to have a direct relationship with God. But Rabbi Bob's religious experience and expression were more indirect, through stories, traditions, rituals, knowledge, and faith. This left me feeling like a Jewish anthropologist, and I wanted more than that.

The rest of the Western religious world offered me the same indirect experience, but with different theologies. I knew my soul's food was elsewhere. Even Taoism wasn't in my destiny. Instead, it was the community of people living for each other that helped make my decision. After much consideration, I decided to become a disciple of the Sikh Guru. Sikh Dharma would become my lifelong path.

I have always been blessed with the ability to commit; discipline is my gift. I stay with the things that I love to do, and I became committed to my new lifestyle. But I needed to practice with fewer distractions from family and friends. An opportunity presented itself when I went to live in a Sikh ashram that also served as a drug rehabilitation program. I moved to Tucson, Arizona, to train as a drug rehabilitation counselor while also experiencing the Sikh lifestyle, all under one roof. It was there, serving the needs of the drug addicted, that I began to live as a Sikh.

After three months of training in Tucson, I returned to Los Angeles as a Sikh—turban, clothing, and all. My experience serving this population helped heal me of some of my own emotional addictions. I returned to Los Angeles to begin a new life, with new disciplines, to help move me toward my destiny. I had developed a consistent disciplined life through years of gymnastics, and now I would attempt to apply that training to the life of devotion.

From Discipline to Disciple

From the word *discipline* comes disciple. Most spiritual disciplines require one to become a disciple of a teacher—that is, a person or personality—this can often lead to disillusion and crises of faith. Eventually we disconnect from the teachings because of the teacher. A sustainable discipline comes from a deep love for the teachings. In this way, our service to the teacher is in the name of the teachings, which in turn serve us. Serving a master honors the discipline and the one who has lived it. When you live it, you embody it. It becomes you.

Most people don't understand the rigorous disciplines of the Sikh path. But to me, they not only define me, but they also serve my destiny. I get up in the morning at about 3:30 to practice my daily discipline, known as *sadhana*, which includes yoga, meditation, and prayer. I love the discipline because it gives me calmness, contentment, and comfort. The discipline becomes self-sustaining when it becomes more fun than work, though it starts out as more work than fun! This has been my experience with several disciplines. Just as I had I studied gymnastics as a child, practicing hours and hours to develop my skills; just as I did with music—now I apply that same enthusiasm to yoga, meditation, singing, prayer, and service.

"The treasure of the Name Nectar, for the sake of which thou hast come into the world, that Nectar is with the Guru. Discard ritual garbs, disguises, cleverness, and duality. With these, the fruit is not obtained. (1) O, my Self, remain in poise and wander not anywhere. Searching outside, thou shalt suffer much pain. The Nectar is in thy heart, at home. Pause."[14]

To succeed at just about anything, you need three things: desire, direction, and discipline. Practice with your heart's desire; allow your desire to fuel your actions in positive ways. My heart's desire is a longing to belong, which most of us share. As I live the Guru's discipline, the Guru embraces me, and what I need in order to succeed comes to me. The discipline works on my ego, refining and redefining it through the practice. My soul's longing, and its connection to the Great Soul, brings ease to the discipline until finally, I am no longer doing the practice, the practice is doing me. This refinement brings its own challenges. For me, the greatest challenge has been maintaining a discipline while sick or injured. The ego wants to do the discipline on its own terms.

During my gymnastic career, I had suffered numerous small injuries. While recovering, I would ask myself why I had been injured. I pondered that question while patiently waiting to heal. But after healing, I wasted little time putting myself at risk again. The risk required a one-pointed focus and brought with it a small taste of oneness, fulfilling that longing to belong, if only for a moment. When I did gymnastics, I was chasing my own ego. When I was sidelined by injury, I became depressed and destructive; my ego was no longer being fed. I was attached to the sport and its disciplines

14 Siri Guru Granth Sahib, Page 598, Guru Nanak Dev Ji

for all the wrong reasons. My gymnastic discipline brought me attention but never gave me fulfillment. I now understand that my subconscious attachments caused me to get injured. The joy of doing something well brought me just a taste of the happiness I longed for. It was like being in the kitchen and smelling the delicious food, but not being able to eat and really enjoy it.

A short time after I moved into the Los Angeles ashram, I badly injured my right elbow while doing some risky gymnastic tricks. This was a serious injury that put me in a cast from my wrist to my shoulder. For the first time in my adult life, I was dependent on others for almost everything. For six weeks, I couldn't drive, dress, wash, or cook for myself without assistance. I recall attending one of Yogi Bhajan's classes right after the injury. When he saw me sitting in class with the cast and sling, he began to laugh boisterously. He never asked what happened but continued laughing. He knew that God had delivered a painful gift to me. It was a profound experience, and I learned what living for each other was all about. While injured, I learned how to receive love and kindness from people I barely knew. Because of my injury, I also got the opportunity to learn to sit and meditate. It was almost a year before I could resume doing handstands and the like. For someone who was always moving, this time was very difficult. To sit daily, repeating God's name, knocking on the door of my own soul, and keeping myself open to listening, required new skills and new disciplines.

Changing my regular practice because of the injury brought me a deeper understanding of my soul's purpose. It was like knocking on the gate of consciousness and hoping something would open. I knocked and knocked, but what I didn't know then was that I was closed. The disciplines were a necessary part of opening up, and as painful as the process was, my love of the disciplines didn't allow me to give up. Now all of my disciplines work together in the constant but joyful struggle of serving my own soul. And yet, even now, meditation remains the most challenging discipline for me. A tool for controlling the mind, I need meditation to heal myself of the need for outside attention. I need to continue to cultivate my own inner awareness. God is always there, but I am not always there.

Meditation has given me the experience of God's attention, which has proven to be far more subtle than applause but much more fulfilling. God's love is the ultimate applause. The real discipline is loving myself as God loves me. The grosser skills of my youth have given way to the subtle disciplines of the breath, alignment, and stillness. Now I know that great thrills lie in the subtle.

Chapter Two

The Master of the Heart

The Guru is the form of God that you can meditate on, imagine, and love.[15]

—Guru Nanak

What guides the human heart toward virtue? Toward piety and purity? What guides our longing to become the image of the divine on Earth? What rules determine these virtues, and what is the path that defines the way to righteous living? Who is our guide to the true heart, and where can we find that guide? The path of the true heart requires a guide who can deliver us to *unisonness* with our self and the one who created us: this guide is a True Guru, the Master of Hearts.

15 From Japji, translation by Guruka Singh Khalsa

It is said that God is everywhere, in everything, and yet we doubt because our senses don't recognize the image and form of the formless. To those who haven't awakened, God is hiding in plain sight. God is watching from within and out, but we can't see Him. Our thinking and our feeling create such a distance from our true selves that we are left deep in doubt, which is a very painful place to live.

I grew up in a culture that was guided by the Christian–Judaic moral code. My early experience of how this moral code was applied was essentially this, people did good things in order to feel better. Feelings guided behavior, and how we felt came from our thinking. So we thought, we felt and we acted, in that order. Feelings of virtue were equated with good behavior. For those who doubted the existence of God, Human Intelligence became the God and superseded everything. Knowledge was all that was needed to succeed in being human. So the motivation was to know more. So, life became: know more, do more, have more, and then enjoy the feelings of success.

The "smartest guys in the room" became the gurus of the secular world, and for those who adhered to this belief system, the holy land was Harvard, Yale, and Princeton. Education and connections were everything: what you knew and who you knew were the guiding principles of success. But in my experience, the more I knew, the darker my mind became. The knowledge I pursued defined my ego, and because of my ego I lived in my head. I had sentenced myself to house arrest. And even though I was already overcrowded with information, all I knew was that I wanted to know more. All of this information didn't lead to wisdom, instead it often led to misguided and confused thinking. Yet squeezed within all of this knowledge and information was a deep longing for my soul. And that longing was enough for me to begin praying for a way out.

By grace my prayers were answered, and my Guru appeared. Without the True Guru I would have remained trapped in the headspace of my ego. Without a True Guru there is no freedom from the cycle of thoughts—1,000 thoughts per wink of the eye. Guru is literally defined as dark to light. The Guru's word, if obeyed, frees us from our thinking. The Guru in Sikh Dharma is the Holy Word that shines and lights the way to the God within our own hearts. The heart is the domain of listening while the head is the domain of thinking. By bowing our heads to the Guru's words we bathe our spirits in songs of God's praise and are liberated from endless thinking and thinking. Obeying the Guru's teachings frees us from the disease of ego so that we can listen, and take the truth to heart and live truthfully. This blessing can only be experienced at the feet of the Guru.[16]

> *Egotism is opposed to the Name of the Lord; the two do not dwell in the same place. In egotism, selfless service cannot be performed, and so the mind goes unfulfilled.*
>
> *O my mind, think of the Lord, and practice the Word of the Guru's Shabad. If you submit to the Hukam of the Lord's Command, you shall meet with the Lord, and then egotism will depart from within. || Pause || Egotism is within all bodies; through egotism, we come to be born. Egotism is utter darkness; in egotism, no one can understand anything.*
>
> *In egotism, devotional worship cannot be performed, and the Hukam of the Lord's Command cannot be understood. In egotism, the soul is in bondage, and the Naam does not come to abide in the mind.*
>
> *O Nanak, meeting with the True Guru, egotism is eliminated, and then, the True One comes to dwell in the mind. Practicing Truth, abiding in Truth, and serving Truth, one is absorbed in the True One.[17]*
>
> —*Guru Amar Das*

16 "Feet of the Guru" is where we bow our head, humbly bringing our ego to divine wisdom
17 Siri Guru Granth Sahib, page 560, Guru Amar Das

True Gurus appear on earth when humanity loses its way. The Bible states that man was created in God's own image, that is, the pure expression of the divine is manifested in the human experience. We were created to express God's fullness. The problem is few of us do. Only such a one who is so pure of heart and full of the divine spirit can bring to earth God's word. By the Grace of God a human becomes a Christ, or a Buddha or a Guru Nanak. By the examples of their love and sacrifice we awaken from our darkness and are called to a spiritual rebirth.

We cannot think our way out of this rebirth, for that we need the true Guru to guide us in our surrender and bring our broken hearts to wholeness. We offer our heads to the true Guru to allow God to enter our hearts and illuminate our minds. And through God's word, humanity can be shown how to live the life we were created for. By Grace I have the Guru's words to define my thinking, the Guru's songs to guide my spirit and the Guru's prayers to assist my conversations with my Creator.

Raj Yog

The True Guru sits on the throne of Raj Yoga and rules the world of form—both subtle and gross. But where do we find this throne, and what is its domain? The throne of Raj Yoga lies in the human heart; its domain is the experience of ease and flow, known as *sahej*, which occurs when we surrender our hearts and our minds and our will to the divine flow of God's will.

An important part of any yoga practice is the experience of comfort. But this comfort is not the same as relaxing on the couch in your living room. This is a deeper comfort that transcends the purely physical. In fact, one of the first principles of Patanjali's sutras[18] is the comfortable seat: asana. We practice kriyas and asana to improve

18   Author of the oldest known yoga texts.

our physical, mental, emotional, and spiritual being. An important part of Kundalini Yoga is the practice of asanas, or postures we take on consciously to make our bodies more resilient, vital, and healthy. At first it may seem to be a contradiction, because asanas aren't comfortable in and of themselves. It takes patience and practice to find that ease within an asana. But pain applied correctly and consciously leads to deeper comfort and physical ease. The idea is to remain calm under the stress of these postures (asanas) so that we can calmly face the stresses of life. As unnecessary tensions subside, the body's circulation increases, as does the health of the tissues. It is a law of the universe that contraction creates expansion. So, too, correct contractions create correct expansions. How we bend and bow, turn and twist, gives form to our devotion. Our bodies become a living prayer—devotion in motion. We need the divine templates of the True Guru to guide our intentions and our contractions, so that we can act faithfully and fulfill our heart's desire to be one with God.

When we learn to sit comfortably, we experience the world within us with more clarity, neutrality, and sensitivity. Within this inner world is the Guru's word and as we listen it can guide our life. The Guru guides us from our dark, shadowed hearts to the light of truth. The light of truth has been with us forever, but our experiences have kept us from recognizing it. We lose the connection to our real self when we attach ourselves to outside influences. By our actions, we move closer to or farther from the light.

The light of the soul illuminates the experience of the true heart which illumines the mind. Just as without sunlight we cannot see the outer world, so too, without the soul's light we cannot clearly see our own inner world. We experience what we call *negative karma* as heaviness, in both our bodies and our minds. Dharma, on the other hand, liberates us from the weight of karma and delivers us to the path of righteousness. We can choose to carry the burden of karma or to be carried by dharma.

Guru is the guide. We take the Guru's words, and we make them our own. We make the Guru's actions our actions. We make the form of the Guru our form. If we choose to be carried by dharma, then the company of other devotees supports us on our path as we absorb the vibration of their song and are inspired by their lives of service and fellowship. Consciousness is not really taught; rather it is caught from those who embody and live it. The company of fellow devotees infects the entire community with greater consciousness. Singing together the songs of the Guru delivers us from our individual consciousness to group consciousness. We experience our oneness and as a *sangat*, a body of people, we become the form of the Guru. We become a body of mastery instead of individual masters. We manifest the Guru's form together.

Once, at a social event, I was introduced to a man who had a great deal of curiosity about me and the way I was dressed; he wanted to know who I was. I told him my name, Guru Prem Singh, and he asked, "How do you become a guru?" I explained that my name meant, "the beloved of the Guru," and that I was not myself a guru. He seemed a bit confused and then asked, "How do you find a guru?" I asked why he wanted one. He explained that his life had become stressful and confused, and he needed a guide to tell him what to do. The word *guru* has become quite common in our culture. We have golf gurus, investment gurus; there is a never-ending parade of gurus.

A guru is commonly understood to have great knowledge of something. But I save the term *True Guru* for that wisdom that can deliver us to God. The Guru doesn't tell us what to do directly in terms of the mundane. For example, the Guru won't tell you where to invest your money but will teach you how to prosper. The Guru won't tell you where to vacation but will guide you to happiness. If you obey the Guru's wisdom, the Guru can guide you to experience your soul and teach you how to live with moral strength and not trade your long-term values for short-term benefits. A relationship with the Guru brings clarity, allowing us to act wisely and make conscious, and hopefully, better choices.

I live by the Guru's words, and my actions reflect the Guru's wisdom. To be a Sikh of the Guru requires clarity in order to walk the path successfully. To achieve success in this relationship, we need three things: the heartfelt desire to belong to the Guru, the intelligence and clarity to understand the Guru's teaching, and the discipline to act on and live the teachings. Another way to look at this is to say we need a formula for faith and fortitude. My relationship with the Guru was only made possible because my spiritual teacher, Yogi Bhajan, worked with me, challenged me, and molded me to successfully relate to the Guru. I was broken down and rebuilt into a man who could fulfill his destiny. Yogi Bhajan often talked about the quality of diamonds, which come from common carbon, but when put under great pressure and the right conditions, a rare event occurs—a raw diamond is created. Then it can be cut, polished, set, and worn. The cut and polished gem-quality diamond allows the light to shine through brilliantly. The goal of the spiritual teacher is to create gem-quality students so that the light of God can be recognized and shared.

The Guru in Context

The Sikh faith began in 1469 with the birth of Nanak. India was suffering from religious persecution; people were being forced to convert to Islam; and the Hindu majority was weighted down by thousands of years of superstitions and a caste system that had long held people captive to a social system that no longer worked. In the midst of all this, Guru Nanak's message, "There is no Hindu and no Muslim, only the one God," was radical. He taught that human life was for realizing God within our own hearts and he believed in the collective, us. Yogi Bhajan summed it up with, "If you cannot see God in All, you cannot see God at all."

Guru Nanak taught that life is for living and realizing truth. Although a man in form, he embodied the light and vibration of God. Guru Nanak's body became the platform from which God Himself spoke and delivered His message through Gurbani, the Guru's Word.

Nanak's light and truth continued through a succession of nine living Sikh Gurus, building a dharma for the coming new age. The Guru's wisdom arrived to prepare humanity for the challenges that the Aquarian Age would bring. The time has now arrived for superstitions to end and realization to begin.

The *Siri Guru Granth Sahib* is the direct wisdom of the ten Sikh Gurus and many other Sufi and Hindu saints; the light of the Guru's wisdom is now imbued in the word, in the form of a Holy Granth, a "whole knot." The essential teachings of the Guru live in this 1,430-page volume. Although to most people, it's just a book, to Sikhs, it is a divine song of God, sung by many tongues. The meditation of sitting and reading, opening it and putting it away, is a subtle dance of devotion that can become the dance of the soul. Yes, it is a book made up of earthly materials; but the words within can inspire and transform even the most mundane tasks to devotion in motion. This book has opened my heart to experience a worthiness I had never known.

"The Shabad Guru is the everlasting word which has the effect of infinity, so man by his nature can grow into reality, cutting through the clouds and storms to become crystal clear to see the path to his destiny."[19]

—*Yogi Bhajan*

The power of the *Siri Guru Granth Sahib* is not in its earthly pages but in its power to unlock and free my spirit. Reading devotedly from its pages unlocks its power. I bow before the Guru as an act of bowing to my True Self, the word within. Though strange to the Western eye, the practice of bowing, along with the other formal gestures surrounding the *Siri Guru Granth Sahib*, is a device that helps unlock our consciousness into a structured, yet free-flowing life of reverence.

Through the Guru's word, light presides in the human heart so that God's light can prevail throughout the world. When we merge with the word, we merge with the Guru. My transformation has been an ongoing process. Each day I awake and offer my head, my ego in service to the True Guru. The word of the Guru presides, and to the best of my ability, I try to obey. I am not perfect, but I do align myself with the Guru each day, and I laugh at my mistakes along the way.

Since I began my relationship with the Guru, I have been blessed by a continuous succession of deeper understandings, becoming more and more aware of myself and my life's purpose. I have recited *Japji Sahib*, Guru Nanak's *Song of the Soul,* thousands of times. These recitations continue to reveal new things to me; with the right attitude, each and every day can seem like reading it for the first

19 From the author's personal notes.

time. The challenge is not to recite it in a rote or mechanical fashion. Keeping the redundant and repetitive from becoming a boring obligation requires a constant and renewed devotion. When I do maintain the proper concentration, my deeper self reveals itself to me. Guru Nanak reminds me that only by deep listening (*sunni-ai*) can I recognize God's play in all things. As I continue to learn to listen more deeply, the words of Nanak penetrate deeper into my being.

If I have any real wisdom, I owe it to the Guru's wisdom. A word recognized is a word illuminated; the greater the recognition, the brighter the illumination. Words that are holy bring us to wholeness and transform us into greater beings. Thus we can better navigate, learn, and grow in the world in which we live.

It is said that our destiny is written on our forehead. By bowing, we reform our patterns and change our thinking. As we become absorbed in the Guru's word, new thought patterns yield new patterns in our brow, and thus a new destiny is written. This rebirth allows us to focus on living, breathing, moving, serving, and acting according to the Guru's teachings.

To be a Sikh is to become a "soul bride of God." The True Word (God) is the "groom," and I, the "bride," sing the Lord's song. My ego is feminine in relationship to the unchanging Great Soul, Mahatma. I have no light of my own; I am just a cold dark moon. But as I turn my face toward God, I become a lighthouse to guide myself and others to the true home in the heart. God lives in the hearts and minds of *Gurmukhs*, or those in whose mind the Guru lives. As the Guru says, "My Soul abides in my heart or rather my Lord abides in my Soul. Now I realize there is no difference between my Soul and my beloved."[20] And as Yogi Bhajan has told us, "A song

20 Siri Guru Granth Sahib, page 1377, Saint Kabir, 15th Century Sufi Saint, 15th Century Sufi Saint

which brings you together as one is the only thing in human nature that brings God, heaven, and earth together, in oneness."[21]

To be able to embody the word and live its truth requires preparation. I was blessed to study with great teachers from the time I was very young. I learned how to obey, serve, love, and excel. Although none of my early teachers were gurus, they provided me with needed expertise. I was a good student when I had respect for the teacher. These early teachers prepared me well for meeting my spiritual teacher, Yogi Bhajan. Although he was not a guru, he deeply embodied the spirit and wisdom of the Guru's teachings and delivered his students to the Guru's feet. Because of his devotion and discipline, he became a *Gurmukh*. Although I served Yogi Bhajan for 30 years, my real devotion was always to the Guru.

A Teacher's Challenge

Realization happens in many stages and levels of refinement. Sometimes the student is blessed by meeting a spiritual teacher. I was blessed in such a way. My spiritual teacher accelerated my relationship with the Guru by offering me numerous challenges. And the Guru brought me through each one. Some challenges were short and humorous, with little pain, and some were long and difficult.

Yogi Bhajan's goal for me and the rest of his students was to make us teachers for the Aquarian Age. I feel most blessed that he succeeded with me. I learned how to be humble and capable of receiving the wisdom of the True Guru. Once you have committed to the Guru, your devotion will be tested. Testing is a part of our growth; tests allow for advances in our realization. I was certainly tested on many accounts, and I am still. With every test, big or small, my reliance on the Guru has proved true; the Guru comes forward to assist and guide me through every obstacle. As Yogi Bhajan has said, "Good

21 ©The Teachings of Yogi Bhajan, Aquarian Wisdom: Yogi Bhajan Everyday 2011

and bad, happy and sad, all is the test of your excellence; love and life, fight and strife, all is the test of your essence."[22]

One of my earlier challenges in my new lifestyle happened the day President Ronald Reagan was shot. Yogi Bhajan asked me to pick up one of his secretaries at the airport. It was about 11 p.m., and I was tired by the time I arrived at Los Angeles International Airport (LAX). In those days, you could pick someone up at the gate. So when I went through a security gate, I was surprised when the metal detector alarm went off. I wondered what could be causing the problem; then I remembered what was in my pocket. Earlier that day I had received a *kirpan* (a knife that Sikh's carry as a symbol of their willingness to defend the innocent). So there I was, taking a large knife out of my jacket pocket, much to the alarm of the airport security officials. I hoped that an apology would be enough and that I could continue on. But that was not to be the case.

Possibly because hours earlier the president barely escaped assassination, or perhaps purely due to my Sikh dress, I was soon in handcuffs. I was arrested for carrying a concealed weapon and taken to the airport police station. I thought to myself that I needed to be focused and remain calm, as I didn't want to do anything to make my situation worse. Mentally I began chanting to Guru Ram Das the 4th Sikh Guru, in part to take my mind off the fact that the handcuffs were on so tight that they cut into my wrists; fear can be a real help when you need to focus. I was taken into the booking station where I was met by the station commander. I stood before him dressed in my white Sikh clothing and turban, with my hands still tightly cuffed behind my back. I made an effort to stand especially straight, as I wanted to look like I didn't belong there. The station commander was holding the kirpan and studying it closely. After a bit of time, he looked up at me and asked what

---

22 From the poem, "The Test," by Yogi Bhajan, the Siri Singh Sahib

I thought was an odd question: "Are you a pacifist?" I thought nobody of his rank could possibly be asking such a question. I began to think that he must be testing me.

The commander continued to question me about who I was, what I did, and so on. I was informed that this was a very serious offense and that if convicted, jail time and a fine were likely. I just stood and breathed and listened for inner guidance. By chance, this was all happening on the eve of my birthday. I thought that mentioning my soon-to-be birthday might get me some sympathy. It didn't. When answering his questions about what I did, I mentioned that I was the gymnastics coach at a local school. I also mentioned that I had attended the University of Southern California and competed in gymnastics there. The commander immediately interrupted, "You were on the gymnastics team at USC?" I assured him I was. He then asked if I knew John "so-and-so"? I replied that John and I were friends through college and that we still kept in touch. It turns out that John was his nephew. What a difference a few words can make! The commander had my handcuffs removed and asked me to sit down. He was now curious how a gymnast from USC could have changed so much. So I told him my story.

As I told him about my involvement with Kundalini Yoga and the Sikh lifestyle, other officers began to wander in and listen to my experiences. The commander and the other officers became very interested in Kundalini Yoga. So I started to share and demonstrate. With my hands free, I didn't waste the opportunity to demonstrate that I was still a gymnast as well as a yogi. I began teaching what became a very impromptu Kundalini Yoga class at the LAX police station. A few moments into the third exercise, the commander said that if I had no outstanding arrest warrants I could go, but not before I answered a few more yoga-related questions. Soon after, they drove me back to the terminal.

By then I was so late, I was sure I had missed my pickup. Much to my surprise, however, the plane was almost two hours late, and I was just on time! The secretary apologized for keeping me out so late. On the drive back from the airport, I recounted what had happened. As I told the tale, the secretary kept telling me what a blessing it had been. I knew she was right. Something about that night felt like a birthday present from the Guru to me.

Another test came as a direct result of my teacher, Yogi Bhajan. He decided that it was time I should be married and that he would find me a wife. Initially, I wasn't comfortable with the thought of an arranged marriage, but I felt guided by my inner Guru to agree. I recognized that my past relationships had all amounted to little. So a matchmaker might be a good idea. I had faith in my teacher and trust in my Guru. At the time, I was feeling burdened by years—or possibly lifetimes—of karma. I was living a lifestyle very different from the one in which I was raised. However, a few months earlier, I had helped rescue a young girl from drowning, which I experienced as a miracle.[23] That near-drowning event created in me a deep sense of gratitude and humility. In the wake of that event, I was willing to accept Yogi Bhajan's request regarding this marriage.

One week after his request, I was married to someone I had only just met. All I knew about her was that she was from France and had come to Los Angeles to study with Yogi Bhajan and to change her life. I am by nature a cautious and deliberate type of person. The idea of making this level of commitment without any due diligence was not what I would typically do. But the next thing I knew, I was taking the vows and planning a life with someone I did not know at all. This marriage ultimately lasted seven years, which is a cycle of consciousness in the teachings of Yogi Bhajan, who says it is possible

23 See page 98 for the story.

to rewrite your destiny in seven years. For me, those seven years turned out to be the greatest transformational period of my life.

As it turned out, it was never meant to be one of those happily-ever-after marriages. What I didn't know at the time of the marriage was that my new wife suffered from some serious eating disorders—anorexia and bulimia. These diseases would come to define the relationship. She ultimately healed herself, but it took seven years. As I became aware of the situation, I sought guidance from all directions. I believed it was my karma to help heal her. After a year of effort, I spoke to Yogi Bhajan about ending the marriage. He was quick to tell me, "You are not getting a divorce." With those words, I began to deeply meditate on why he wanted me to suffer along with her. It was a major crisis in my faith. What should I do? I felt I had a no graceful way out, so I went within. I began what I call my "monk" period. While I became her caretaker, I also began a deep adventure within myself.

I began to listen closely to my inner voice. We were living in the ashram with eight other people. No one really understood what I was going through, mostly because I kept as much as possible from them. I hid what I could and began to take care of myself. I built my own room, so I could have some privacy, a place to just be. It also served as a music room for myself. In the beginning, it was just for playing guitar and piano; but over time, I started to collect more instruments. Practicing kept me occupied in my free time and provided me with an escape from the stress. This worked well enough while at home. I also put a lot of effort into teaching yoga and building my healing practice of neural-skeletal posture therapy.

Yogi Bhajan knew I was suffering at home, but he helped keep me busy by sending me clients. He also allowed me the privilege of working on him, so I was able to talk to him regularly. However, he continued to insist that I stay married. After four years of "the marriage," I received a call from Yogi Bhajan to visit. I expected to just give him a treatment. But upon my arrival, he asked, "Are you still married to that woman?" Before I could answer, he said, "I would have divorced her years ago." I was speechless!

He spoke to me then, and his words remain priceless. He let me know he had been aware of how difficult the situation had been. Then he asked me this: "As a personal favor to me, stay with her a bit longer until she becomes stable; then it will be over." He went on to say that he would start working with the both of us daily. It took another three years before she became free of the disease. Two things allowed me to survive this period. First of all, I began to build a recording studio. I spent nearly all of my free time studying the science of recording. When things seemed impossible at home, a soothing voice inside my heart would say, "Buy yourself some more equipment." Each piece of recording gear required a significant amount of time to learn. I became compulsive and learned everything I could about recording. Second, I witnessed my wife's miraculous healing under Yogi Bhajan's guidance. She agreed to spend eight hours every day sitting in the Guru Ram Das Ashram, practicing *tablas* (Indian Drums). She would sit at the back of the ashram and practice for hours on end. Yogiji would regularly check up on her, as she continued in this manner almost every day for two years. The "tabla kriya" ultimately freed her from her disease. Our marriage didn't start as a relationship of love and affection, and it didn't end as one either. Instead, it served a very different purpose—one of personal transformation. It brought me to a profound state of listening, and it brought her to a real and lasting healing. I got through it all because I learned to listen.

After seven years of marriage, I was walking to the Gurdwara on a Sunday morning. As I turned the corner, I noticed Yogi Bhajan walking by himself, which is something he almost never did. There he was, by himself, walking toward me; I waited for him so that we could walk the last block together. A few steps after we met, he stopped and turned to me and said, "I have annulled the marriage." It was finally over! What had felt like a seven-year kriya was finally ending, as if he had said, "Inhale," and I could finally put my arms down.

As we continued walking, Yogi Bhajan stopped me a second time and said, "We are going to start a music business." I hadn't told him about my hobby, but a few days later he began sending me his poems and asked that I put them to music. He also insisted that I use one of his administrative secretaries named Nirinjan Kaur to sing on the recordings. Until that time, I had not done any real song writing. But as I looked at his inspiring poetry, I began to hear the music. Something inside me unlocked, and I could hear things that I'd never heard before. All together I recorded about 33 of his poems and mantras. Yogi Bhajan used the recordings extensively, and I began to sell what were then cassette tapes, and later CDs. A small business was born, which continues to prosper even today.

My whole life—and those seven years in particular—prepared me well for my future and for the life I live today. I am now happily married with two beautiful children. I still practice listening in order to remain prepared for the life ahead. But I have faith in my teacher and trust in my Guru that all is well. "There is no good or bad, thinking makes it so."[24]

---

24 Yogi Bhajan paraphrasing from Shakespeare, *Hamlet Act 2, scene 2*

Chapter Three

Surrender:
The Life of the Devotee

Many religions proclaim to be the only true path to God. Yet, if they all claim to be the only way, then how do we know what to bow to? Whose formula really works? How do we find the teachings that are worthy of our surrender? And why would we want to surrender in the first place? As Westerners, we often equate surrender with defeat or collapse. If we surrender, it means we're falling apart, right? Actually the path of wisdom guides us to surrender what's no longer needed and to receive what serves us. A good place to begin surrendering is in our relationship to the ego.

Before we can begin the search, we, the seekers, must be in the right relationship with the ego. The ego must be tempered before the search begins. Life, with all its ups and downs, is probably the single greatest tempering agent. We are fired by the trials of life and love, and we are reformed, changed into something, hopefully, a little wiser and a little more tolerant. We are humbled. My favorite definition of *humility* is "to become approachable." When we are humbled, we become open-hearted, ready to recognize and receive our true teacher.

The student finds the teacher, not the other way around. We receive the teacher we've earned so that we can fulfill the destiny written for us—or the one we hope to write. But first we must experience the longing for a teacher, and humility is the key. We can either humble ourselves or be humiliated—either way, we bow; we listen. If given the choice, it is better to learn from a teacher than from time and space. We have a choice: to learn by grace or to learn from suffering; to surrender and listen or to keep thinking and managing and struggling until time and space teaches us.

We have no real power other than the choices we make. When we listen to the word of the Guru as it is read or recited, we hear it and hopefully take it to heart. But when we hear the word of the Guru from within, we can accept the word and hopefully live it. This is a deep listening of the heart, which leads to acts of faith and ultimate surrender. Faith in the Guru's word is required before heartfelt acceptance and surrender can be realized. And before faith can be realized, we need the truth. However, the truth is hidden from our five physical senses and is realized only by a sixth sense— intuition. Deep intuition is awakened as we listen and act in faith.

Acting in faith requires obedience—that is, listening to our inner voice and agreeing to agree. When we listen and heed the inner voice of the Guru, that's true surrender. The command of the Guru is known as *hukam*, or an order from God. Often misunderstood as just another list of moral codes and ethics, *hukam* is instead an act of acceptance of what is—Sat Nam, the True Name. If you accept the word of the Guru as the word of God, then the goal is to follow it and live it. Surrendering to the *hukam* of God's word requires faith. But faith in what? Faith in wisdom, which speaks of the truth in everything. The Guru presents the truths of God within the laws of nature, even though sometimes God's word can transcend the laws of nature. In the Old Testament of the Bible, the Red Sea parted for Moses and his people. Whether this was an act of God transcending nature doesn't really matter. Faith in the story as a testament of truth—not fact—is what matters. The story is a device to deliver our faith to fulfillment. The stories about people living or being tested by truth change every time they are told; the facts are constantly being altered. And yet, the truth within the story remains unchanged.

Faith and surrender are close kin. In order to have faith, we must surrender doubt. Doubt casts its shadow on the heart's light of truth. We need intelligence to choose our teachers carefully, and then we need the courage to surrender with faith to those teachings. When we live in acceptance and have the courage to face the facts, we can begin to live them with faith and fortitude. When we live by the word, in obedience to *hukam*, we experience *sahej*, or the ease that comes from surrender to the will of God.

What started more than 500 years ago with the birth of Nanak eventually grew into a *dharma*, a path of righteous living. This way of living sets out to help conquer man's fear of death. We are so attached to our ego identity that we run from death; but we can't run from our fear of death, because it chases after us. By living as this separate ego identity, we remain separated from our True Self.

*Ek Ong Kaar, Sat Nam, Karta Purkh, Nirbhao, Nirvair, Akal
Moorat, Ajoonee, Saibhang, Gurprasad, Jaap. Aad Sach,
Jugaad Sach, Haibhee Sach, Nanak Hosee Bhee Sach*
—*Guru Nanak*

Described by Guru Nanak in the *Mul*, or Root Mantra, of the *Siri
Guru Granth Sahib*, the True Self is expressed in *Ek Ong Kar*—
One Creator, creating. This creation is happening continuously in
all of us and in everything. *Sat Nam*, the creation, you and me
are all formed out of truth. We are formed from the formless.
Karta Purakh—from the light of truth, the creation moves and
does everything. Truth is the power that gives us our life and our
living. We move in ways both large and small, but what guides our
movement is *nirbhao* and *nirvair*. The creator projects his creativity
and moves without fear or anger, and we share this identity and
destiny. It is our challenge to live it. *Akaal moorat* means "deathless
personified." We do not acknowledge death as our end. Our soul
was neither created nor can it be destroyed; it is deathless.

The Latin word for *exhale* is *experio*, which actually means "death"
or expire." Our fear of death weakens us from exhaling into our
true home—the heart center. Because breathing is both emotional
and physical, fear of death alters both movement and feelings. An
intelligent and conscious exhale delivers us back to our heart center.
If we are deathless, then we are living in our true identity, and we
are birthless, or *ajoonee*, our immortal self. It cannot die because it
was not born. There is no beginning or end to our consciousness.
Humans have no bottom and no top; in this way, we mirror the
infinite, limitless nature of the Creator. Just as the worst human
behavior could still get worse, so too when you think you have seen
the greatest saint, you find there is still room for improvement. Why
is this? It is answered by the word *saibhang, self-existent*. The light
of God has always existed, just as the light of our souls has always

existed and always will. Our ego-based behavior casts shadows over the light of the soul, and we live in the illusion of darkness. As we transcend the ego, however, we begin to recognize the light by remembering that God's name was true in the beginning, true through all ages, true right now, and always true: *Aad Sach, Jugaad Sach, Haibhee Sach, Naanak Hosee Bhee Sach.*

All of creation adheres to G.O.D.: Generation, Organization, and Destruction or Deliverer. From the formless, forms are constantly being generated, given shape and purpose, and then returned and recycled, again and again. Let's look at gravity as an example. No scientist can tell us exactly what gravity is; science can only explain its effects. Nor can scientists explain the original cause that created the universe—that is, how something came from nothing. Simply stated, gravity makes things move. Every form, subtle or gross, has a relationship to everything around it, making things in and around it move. Gravity does not operate in a predestined manner. All that is determined is that "all things come from God and all things go to God."

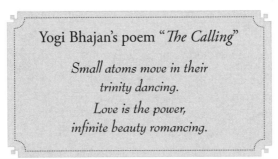

Yogi Bhajan's poem *"The Calling"*

*Small atoms move in their
trinity dancing.
Love is the power,
infinite beauty romancing.*

God's love is the power that makes things move, take form, and return to the formless. With the True Guru's guidance, we can flow on the path of dharma, or we can suffer on the path of karma.

Developing our intelligence to serve the heart's wisdom is paramount. We must recognize that this human body was designed to be conscious and conscientious, to make wise choices and to live truthfully. In this way, we serve our own destiny with renewed faith and fortitude. Thinking, in itself, does not bring us any closer to our souls, but it can become a tool that ultimately teaches us to bow. And the act of bowing aligns our bodies and our minds with our surrender to our soul, where we can know *sahej*—ease—and live by listening—*sunni-ai*—tuned into the song of our soul.

We often contract and expand as an expression of our egos. But we can also contract and expand as an expression of sacrifice or surrender. We can learn to use the muscles of the sacrum to help create wholeness—holiness—in the body. The sacred contraction of the pelvic muscles establish the foundation for correct and balanced expansion of the physical body. This is the foundation of divine alignment. At one time what was understood to be sacred became forbidden. The science of the sacred, especially regarding sexuality and creativity, was lost or hidden. As the sacred nature of the human experience became more and more obscured by religion and other social strictures, as the creativity and sexuality of human nature was deemed forbidden, humans became more and more disconnected from their own divinity. We lost the ability to experience the sacred. Sacred acts require contraction, which, by universal law, creates expansion, which is divine. This is the polarity that we balance with each and every breath.[25]

Sometimes, however, sacredness is put upon us and feels like a burden, as my prior marriage did. We are often forced by circumstances to contract. But if we can humbly receive this burden, it becomes a bridge to our own surrender and a deeper relationship to our own soul's destiny. With this relationship, we become God's instrument on Earth. God needs us to sing his song, play his rhythm, and dance to his drum. Another line from

---

25 See Bowing Jaap Sahib on page 158 for a practice of surrender, contraction and expansion.

a poem by Yogi Bhajan speaks to this: "Live as you're destined, surrender the tension, the healings in place, call on His Grace, and follow the faith." We can surrender the unnecessary tension so that circumstances, as gifts of the Guru and of God, come to serve us. In this way, the servant becomes the master. To surrender is to allow God to serve us through his love. Common are those who love God, but rare is the one who is truly open to receiving and experiencing God's love. With the True Guru's guidance, we can surrender to the sacred and live in the *sahej*.

God can do all but one thing—create another God. God can expand or contract only through his creation. Our surrender allows God to love himself and to know the devotion of the devotee.

Sleep & the Practice of Surrender

"Death is a good sleep."
—Yogi Bhajan

For me, going to sleep is the practice of letting go to die. Ideally thinking ends, and bliss begins. The deeper you sleep, the less sleep you need. Some people spend eight to ten hours in bed getting poor, unrestful sleep. While others are able to sleep four to six hours of very deep sleep and awaken fully restored. I believe the deeper the sleep, the more we let go of our body, mind, and spirit into the protection of our Creator.

When I was a very young child, I had a basic phobia about sleep, which came from my fear of death. I recall asking my father about what happens when you die. He told me, "It's like sleeping without dreams and you disappear forever." This terrified me, and yet it did me a great favor. I refused to believe that I could go from consciousness to insignificance. My fear of death made me pray, and prayer is what sustained me, even at four years old. My father, however, had gone through the transformation of facing death many times during World War II and had arrived at a place where death represented peace from his own ego; he believed there was only the body and mind. For him, death negated his existence; and to him, that was peace.

I believe my father was missing a piece of the puzzle that my years of faith and practice have led me to understand. The physical body ends with death as it breaks down into its base elements. The mind also leaves and dissolves into the subtle elements, thus ending the gross ego. But the soul remains with the history of your life, encoded in what is known as the subtle body. The subtle vibrations surrounding the soul carry the experiences of this and countless other lifetimes.

At four, I was afraid of the ego dying, but now I pray for it to die. Allowing the ego to die requires a True Guru. Yet before the ego can die, it needs to help teach you how to live. That is why the ego is both the disease and the cure. My fear of dying was assuaged when I began to hear a reassuring voice within, promising me that I would never disappear. At a very young age, I often tried to remember what my existence was like before I was born. I knew there was more than this body-mind, yet still I was very afraid. This began my secret life of prayer—a secret that I kept from my family. My prayer before bedtime was usually answered by the soothing voice, which said that I could let go and go to sleep.

A good night's sleep is possibly the greatest luxury in life. What people will do to get a good night's rest is both very imaginative and sad. I know people who *have spent more on a mattress than most people spend on a new car. Yet they still find restful sleep difficult to experience. The body and mind require sleep to rest and repair. Many of our bodies' restoration activities only occur while we are sleeping.*

In the United States, about 30 percent of the adult population suffers from chronic sleep difficulties. The world of pharmacology offers many different sleep aids, with Ambien being the most popular. I'm not against its use for occasional sleep problems, but the problem is that Ambien—and other similar prescription medications—are often abused in our increasingly challenged efforts to fall and stay asleep.

The problem is that we go to sleep to relax instead of relaxing to go to sleep. Parents raising children know that you don't just send a four year old to bed; there usually exists a bedtime routine, for the purpose of relaxing, to fall asleep. The child's bedtime routine often includes a warm drink, such as milk or herbal tea, followed by a warm bath or shower; then it's into bed but not to sleep. What usually follows is cuddling, bedtime stories, and hopefully a goodnight prayer. On a deeper level, this routine is the basic training needed to conquer our fear of death. As parents, my wife and I tried to make our children feel safe and secure in their beds. We taught our children from birth to trust their souls to God and Guru. This would allow them to let go of their bodies and minds and easily fall asleep.

Letting go is the most challenging of skills. The twelve-step programs have a saying: "Let go and let God." And that is the secret to sleep! But it is easier said than done. It's difficult enough to relax the muscles, but what about the mind? Relaxation is the active process of turning off the unnecessary tension, so you can feel the hand of God guide you. In this case, relaxation guides us to release our bodies and minds into sleep, which is the biggest challenge to successful sleeping.

The Ten Sikh Guru's made great efforts to bring courage and understanding to our relationship with death. I have learned from the Guru's teachings that the right attitude toward sleep can heal us from the fear of death. The Gurus also taught that we must relax to go to sleep. To that end, they provided a sleep meditation that is the equivalent of giving ourselves the last rites. These "last rites," known as Kirtan Sohila, are to be done every night before sleep. Kirtan Sohila is also recited at the time of death and as part of the Sikh funeral service.

For me, going to sleep is part of a bigger daily discipline, my daily sadhana. Ben Franklin said it best: "Early to bed, early to rise, makes a man healthy, wealthy and wise." How I approach sleep influences how I sleep, as well as my ability to get up very early. My early to rise includes my pre-sadhana: After waking up at around 3:30 a.m., I acknowledge that I am still in my body and that everything works. I go downstairs to boil some water. I brush my teeth, including the back of my tongue, to clean out the bacteria that gathered at night. I then massage my skin with almond oil and take a cold shower. In the cold shower, I usually do Breath of Fire while massaging myself. After I get out, I briskly rub my body as I dry off. After that I get dressed and go downstairs, prepare my green tea, and begin to recite Japji Sahib, the Song of the Soul. Then I practice Kundalini Yoga while listening to Jaap Sahib for about 30 minutes. After yoga, I begin the Aquarian meditations, which includes seven mantras that last about an hour (see below). I am then finally off to Gurdwara for kirtan (devotional singing) prayers and a reading from the Siri Guru Granth Sahib. Some days I join the group sadhana at Yoga West. Or if I am traveling, I may join a local group. That is my basic sadhana.

At the end of the day, one of my single greatest pleasures is to play devotional music on guitar or piano, as this is my favorite way to relax at home—or just about anywhere.

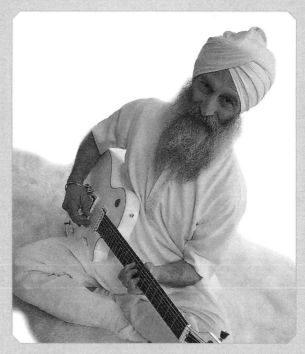

My playlist includes occasional interludes from my past—the songbook and soundtrack of my earlier life. Following that, I usually take a hot shower or bath and prepare for sleep, by which time, my wife is doing her bedtime meditations. My day ends with Kirtan Sohila, which is especially nice when Simran, my wife sings, because she does it so well. Sometimes, for a change, I'll accompany her on guitar; other times, I'll do a specific meditation before sleep as well.

This recitation, which in itself is a meditation, is to be done only in the later afternoon or evening; it doesn't have to be done right before bed.

Kirtan Sohila: Evening Prayer[26]

Raag Gauri Melah Pela
(1st Guru Nanak)

In that house where holy men dwell ever on the lord
reciting his name,
in that house meditate on him and joyously sing his praises,
Yes, sing the praises of the Lord the fearless one,
I would give my life
for that song which imparts the peace eternal.
Everyday the Lord is watching all his beings, the great giver,
looks to the needs of all creatures
His gifts are beyond all measure; then how may
one describe the giver?
The day of marriage of the soul bride with her Lord has dawned,
Oh friends, my friends pour the oil of love down on the threshold
and give me
all of your blessings, that I may know a perfect
union with my Lord.
This call is being sent to all, sent to all homes each day,
so forget not the one who calls, the one who calls each day.
Oh, Nanak, the day is drawing near for everyone.

26 A version of Kirtan Sohila with Simran Kaur Khalsa is available at
www.kundaliniresearchinstitute.org to listen or download and practice at home.

Raag Asa Guru Nanak

*There are six systems and six teachers and
six are their different teachings,
but the teacher of all is the one Lord who meets
a man in so many forms.
One should practice those teachings where his praises
are in some way sung,
then one will gain honor.
There is but one sun which runs through the seconds,
minutes, and hours,
the solar and lunar days, the changing seasons of the year.
Just so there is but one God from whom come
all the variety of forms.*

Raag Dhnasi Guru Nanak

The sky is the azure salver, the sun and moon
are thy lamps, the stars are thy
scattered pearls, the sandal forests thy incense,
and the breeze is thy fan.
These along with the flowers of vegetation
are laid as offerings at thy feet.
Oh, destroyer of fear, what other worship can be compared
to nature's own festival
of lights while the divine music resounds within.
Thousand are thine eyes and yet thou hast no eyes.
Thousand are thy forms and yet thou hast no form.
Thousand are thy lotus feet and yet thou hast no feet.
Thousand are thy noses to smell and yet thou hast no nose.
I am enchanted with thy play; it is the light which lives
in every heart and thy
light which illumines every soul.
Whatever is pleasing to thee, that is the true worship.
My soul yearns for the honey of thy lotus feet.
Night and day I am a thirst for thee, I am like that bird
who cries "peo, peo,"
waiting to receive the drop of water, which is the nectar of thy
kindness so that I may live in the ecstasy of thy name.

Raag Guri Purbhi Guru Ram Das

This human body is filled with the passions of lust and anger,
but in the presence of the saints I am freed from their bonds.
My last life's Karma has led me to the true Guru,
and by his kindness my
heart has obtained a permanent place
in the Lord's sanctuary of Love.
Make a salutation before the saints—that is an act of piety,
bow deeply before them—this brings great virtue.
The Maya worshipers, stuck by the thorn of pride,
do not know the taste of the Lord's nectar; as they
walk away from God, that thorn pierces deeper
and the greater is their suffering until they bring
death upon themselves.
God's slaves live ever in his name; yes they have broken the
fear of birth and death, for they have found God, the Eternal
and they are honored through all the universes and worlds.
I am meek and lowly but I belong to thee, oh Lord,
save me for thou art greatest of the great!
Thy name is slave Nanak's only support and in thy Name
he has found perfect peace.

Raag Purbi Guru Arjan

Listen, my friends, I beg of you.
Now is the time to serve the saints, and in earning merit
here you will live in bliss forever.
Each night and day brings this life closer to its dreaded end,
so go and search out the Guru and settle your account.
This world is enveloped in evil and duality.
That man alone whom God awakens to the nectar of his Name
comes to realize the teachings of the indescribable Lord.
Use this life to achieve that purpose for which it
was given and through the Guru
God will come to live with you.
Your soul will return to its true home, finding perfect peace,
and this round of
births and deaths shall cease.
Oh Lord, who knows the inner most reaches of our hearts and
who gives to each the fruits of their actions,
fulfill also the desire of my mind.
Nanak, thy slave, wants no other happiness than this—
that he may become the dust under the feet of thy saints.

Breath & Bones

Getting to Sleep

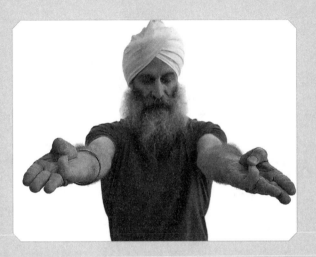

In addition to my evening prayers, I have found this meditation helps clear the subconscious, which allows for a more productive and restful sleep. To do this meditation, sit in any seated position you enjoy. Tune in with the Adi Mantra (see page 56): Ong Namo Guru Dev Namo. Bring your spine into proper alignment. Extend your arms straight out in front of you, parallel to the ground with the palms up. Hook the thumbs over the "mercury finger"— the little finger. Keep the other fingers straight and the arms stretched out. Gaze at the Third Eye and begin to chant a long Wahe Guru. Do this for a maximum of 11 minutes; then rest. If you wish, you can then repeat it once more for another 11 minutes or less.

Sometimes if I'm really unable to fall asleep, I'll do bridge pose to help my nervous system relax. Afterward, I do my own personal prayers and then to sleep.

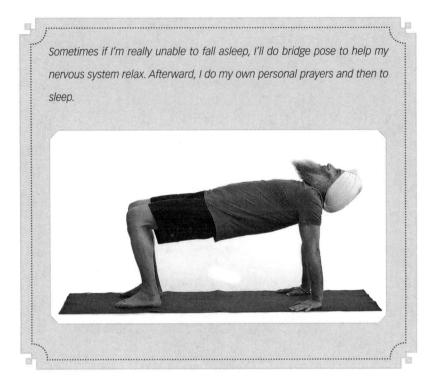

Chapter Four

Temples and Templates

It has been said that the body is the temple of the soul. The human mind and body are simply the vehicles through which we experience our soul and our humanity. The Bible states that we are created in the image of God, and other religious traditions concur. The human experience is unique among sentient beings in that the human body gives us the capacity to see and know God. It is our destiny to merge in His identity and become His form. We can all somewhat relate to the concept of merging in the identity of God; but what would it mean to become the form of God, a temple of divine consciousness?

Let's begin at the beginning by looking at our terms—*temple* and *template*. A template is usually thought of as a device to guide the accuracy of forms. Templates are necessary to make sure lines are straight, symmetry is maintained, and directions are accurate. But the origins of the word template come from an older definition, meaning the "form of the temple." If we think of the body as a temple of the soul, then its templates are the geometry of consciousness, self-awareness, and applied intelligence. These seats of awareness abide within the human form—the body—which is made up of at least thirty trillion cells dancing throughout our system. Combined with the power of gravity, these dancing cells define our form. The nature of form demands that it move, change, and ultimately be destroyed.

Do we move toward our destiny or toward our fate? Do we lose our innocence or regain our purity? Do we face death with courage or fear? Do we live a life based on consciousness or one based on emotions and commotions? A life guided by feelings and emotions leads to duality. I once heard Yogi Bhajan say, "Look for the trinities; they will lead to balance. Avoid dualities; they will lead to suffering."[27] In yogic philosophy, the One became two, two became three, and from the three came everything—the multiplicity of the entire universe. The number three represents the qualities of the manifested universe—G.O.D., or Generator, Organizer and Destroyer or Deliverer. It represents a harmony and a balance, a natural movement within the cycle of life.

According to Yogi Bhajan, "Devotion is the polarity of emotion."[28] Most of us have to experience some level of suffering before we're willing to move toward devotion. How much is enough is different for each of us. As we move from emotion to devotion, as we use the principle of the trinity—balance—to guide our experiences, we move beyond duality toward unity. Therefore, a life of devotion leads to oneness—*pratyahar*—embodied in the mantra *Ang Sang Wahe Guru*, which describes our cells dancing in the light of God's

27 From the personal notes of the author.
28 © The Teachings of Yogi Bhajan, July 5, 1982

name. This is the state of balance in the human experience where we no longer identify ourselves by our suffering. Through *pratyahar*, a state of balance, we can tracend the limitations experienced through the five physical senses. But how do we teach these myriad intelligences, trillions of individual cells, to bow, to surrender, and to entrain in harmony with one another and with the Higher Self? In short, how do we teach them to recognize the Master? We need templates to guide our development—templates that represent the qualities of the divine in the form of a Guru.

Through the practice of Kundalini Yoga, we can develop, strengthen, and refine the *shakti* energy, the primal force of creativity and balance. Asanas and kriyas build the foundation for the "comfortable seat," which is the seat of the divine within our hearts—the throne of Raj Yoga. Singing the Guru's hymns causes a cellular frequency to shift, which allows the body to adopt the behavior of the Guru. We walk, talk, move, sing, dance, fight, love, and so on like the Guru. We are not the Guru; but like the moon reflects the Sun's light, we reflect the light of the Guru. With the Guru's template, we become *Gurmukhs*, liberated from time and space. We live in such a way that all thought and action are sacred; this is the dedicated life wherein we become the living principle of the Guru's discipline.

The soul has an innate longing to belong to the infinite. However, that longing can take us in different directions: We can either conform to the emotional, commotional world of our peers and family pressures, or transform and become the very likeness of God. It's our choice. The Guru gives us the template, and through the Guru's guidance, we become the form of the formless. In my early days of transformation, I felt deformed. I was ruled by my emotions and feelings and suffered consequences from the limitations they brought. Consciousness had been pushed aside because of the need for emotional satisfaction. I needed to change, but there was so much misinformation. What and who could I trust? How could I begin to define the right action for myself or others? What path should I take? These were the questions that vexed me—and yet the answers were within me all along.

When we practice Kundalini Yoga, we begin with the mantra *Ong Namo Guru Dev Namo*. Namo means I bow, Guru Dev is that transparent Guru that is within and around us in every moment; it is that moment of inspiration that we have all experienced at least once in our lives.

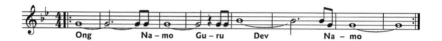

As I began to conform to the Guru's form, the Guru's template, I learned to trust that inner voice, my inner teacher, and began to be guided by the light from within.

The One Minute Breath

My practice of sunni-ai, or inner listening, began with listening as my breath guided the movements of my yoga practice. Hearing Sat on the inhale and Nam on the exhale began to make me feel that the spirit was moving me. Thirty-five years later, I'm still listening, but now I inhale light and love as I vibrate Sat and exhale darkness and doubt as I consolidate the virtues with the sound of Nam. This is the practice of becoming wholehearted—that is, the broken bits of my virtues and vices are refined and then defined by consciously exhaling Nam. The wholeness of my gracefully mended heart becomes holiness, which guides my form with the inhaled sound of Sat. The expanding Sat, or truth, brings to me new light and life. Regardless of the kriya or asana, my practice of deep listening becomes a dynamic prayer, a moving meditation.

A pranayam, or breath meditation, that I often enjoy is called One Minute Breath. Begin by tuning in. The breath cycle is divided into three parts: inhale for 20 seconds, hold for 20 seconds, and exhale for 20 seconds. If 20 seconds is too long, reduce the times but keep each part equal.

It is important to sit up straight with the sit bones properly connected to the ground. A properly applied Mulbandh,[29] correctly contracting the muscles of the navel, sex organ, and anus, allows us to accelerate our development. Correct alignment assists in expanding the back body as well as the chest. Imagine light spreading over the back of the body, like the moon being illuminated by the sun. The back is considered the moon side of the body, and the front, the sun side. This visualization can help develop your inner light. Try this meditation for 11 minutes or longer; it will bring you inner strength, vitality, and greater intuition.

---

29 For a more detailed description of Mulbandh, Uddiyana Bandh, and how to practice Asana's with ease, see Guru Prem's other books, *Divine Alignment & The Heart Rules*

Intuitive Listening: The Template for the Aquarian Age

We live in an age of information overload. But information isn't necessarily truth or wisdom. We have to learn discernment and humility in order to come to the truth, which is often hidden in plain sight. The Guru says, "Truth (God) is like sugar scattered in the sand."[30] If we approach it like an elephant, we suffer as we eat the sand mixed with the sugar. The Guru's advice was to become like an ant, small and humble; this is the way to partake of truth. In the same way, Yogi Bhajan said, "All lives in small." The ego has to become small for the soul to shine. As long as our ego is in the way, we can never feel the soul's infinite source of light and become transformed through our own inner wisdom. The ego is loud; the soul is subtle. As I have grown older, I have learned to experience the thrill of the subtle. Maturity brings with it a radical shift in priorities: Little becomes big, and big becomes small. Now when I bow my head, I receive the fruits of surrender—wisdom, equanimity, and peace.

Other traditions have their own templates, or symbols that inform the life of a devotee. When a Christian wears the crucifix, is it because there is some special power in the wood or the metal? Is there some unique power in the image of Jesus? No, the power isn't in the physical symbol itself; the power is in the heart of the one who wears it, the one who cares for it. The power is in the mind of the devotee. The power of symbols lives within us. If we have faith, symbols have the power to influence our behavior. They have the power to change our minds.

I personally use symbols throughout my life to guide me to my destiny. Pictures and statues throughout my home symbolize what I believe in and what I want to become. My house is the temple

---

30 Siri Guru Granth Sahib, page 972, line 10, Saint Kabir, 15th Century Sufi Saint

of my home life. It is sacred, yet cozy and comfortable. Although I don't personally identify myself as a Buddhist, I have a statue of the Buddha in my backyard. When I see that statue, I take to heart, the peace, serenity, harmony, and grace that it represents. The statue is a device to help find these qualities inside myself. However, it would become idolatry if I were to believe that power resides in the statue.

In addition, I decorate myself with different symbols. For example, I represent myself as consciously as I can through my clothing. I wear white as a symbol of purity and as a technology to increase my auric field. The color white communicates to the world that I'm on a journey toward the pure heart, while my expanded aura lets people know that I'm available for service. I also wear a turban, because the head that serves the True Heart is worthy of being crowned. I wear the symbols of a king, a Raj Yogi, to help me better serve the world. I wear a steel bracelet on my wrist to remind me to whom I belong, so that my work and my actions are righteous. I wear a small wooden comb in my hair to remind myself of the importance of being clean and that my long hair serves my consciousness and my energy as a householder. I also carry a small symbolic sword to indicate my commitment to defend the innocent and the helpless. This small sword unlocks my courage and gives me the capacity to sacrifice myself, if necessary, to defend the defenseless. I also wear *kacheras*, a type of underwear that helps keep my creative energies in alignment with serving the Creator. I dress the part, and the world holds me to the standard that I hold for myself.

Symbols and templates such as these are devices that serve our consciousness. They establish the patterns that the soul uses to transform the body and mind into the divine on Earth—to be one with the God in service of the Guru. We can want to be great, wise, and full of virtue, but without a plan, it's just a fantasy. To succeed, we must have the heartfelt desire combined with the correct direction and discipline; two out of three will fail. Kundalini Yoga is the science of angles and triangles. The angles represent the structure of the temple—how we structure our lives, our behavior patterns, and our bodies. The triangles represent the qualities of energy that flow and circulate within us. Understanding the templates of inner virtue requires recognizing the forms they become. Virtues of the True Heart manifest as harmony, balance, and beauty. Become as good as you look. As you act in virtue, as you cultivate discipline, as you grow in wisdom, you become more beautiful. And your body shows this beauty, from the alignment of your a spine, to the smiles on your face.

The templates of truth are best described in the last pauri of Japji Sahib.

Japji's 38th Pauri by Guru Nanak

Let self-control be the furnace, and patience the goldsmith.
Let understanding be the anvil, and spiritual wisdom the tools.
With the Fear of God as the bellows, fan the flames of tapas, the body's inner heat. In the crucible of love, melt the Nectar of the Name, and mint the True Coin of the Shabad, the Word of God. Such is the karma of those upon whom He has cast His glance of Grace. O Nanak, the Merciful Lord, by His Grace, uplifts and exalts them. || 38 ||

This pauri describes the essence of alchemy, the philosopher's stone that is spoken of in many traditions. Let's look at it line by line:

꧁ *Make continence your furnace and patience your goldsmith.*[31]

This line speaks of leadlike consciousness turned into the heart of gold. Making continence your furnace refers to taking the heat of uncontrolled passions and turning them into compassion. This heat is the basis of transformation, but it can also burn you. The patience of a goldsmith refers to the fine, and often slow, fashioning of a valuable raw material to bring out its beauty. The heart of gold must be patiently fashioned into a majestic work of art.

꧁ *Make understanding your anvil and Divine Knowledge your tools.*

To stand under brings understanding. We become solid and firm through the knowledge gathered by humbly seeking the truth. The anvil's strength and resilience, along with its smooth surface, easily accept the strikes and pressures of the goldsmith's tools. These are the tools of transformation in the forming of the conscious human being.

꧁ *With the Fear of God as the bellows, fan the flames of* tapas, *the body's inner heat.*

An old saying from the Bible says, "Fear of God is the beginning of Wisdom."[32] This fear is special because it is the fear of being disconnected from the love of God. All other fears are to be transcended. Breath is the bellows that fan the flames of transformation. With each inhale, we fan the flames of God's love and compassion and then exhale into the heart, the home of the True Guru.

---

31 Translation by Dr. Sant Singh Khalsa
32 Proverbs 1:7

> *In the crucible of love, melt the Nectar of the Name.*

A crucible can hold smelted metals of a very high heat while maintaining its own integrity. The crucible referred to here is the human heart, which has been tested by obedience and service. A tempered heart is capable of receiving the nectar of bliss. Because of love, the name of God, recited again and again with such devotion, melts away the separation between God and humankind.

> *And mint the True Coin of the Shabad, the Word of God.*

The word unspoken comes to life by the breath and becomes the vibration and the form of the God-man. All of the ingredients are there, and the word is forged into the divine form.

> *Such is the karma of those upon whom He has cast His glance of Grace.*

Our actions either draw God to us or give distance. As we serve the True Guru and become the crucible of his teachings, we are defined, refined, and cast into form; we are blessed by God's glance of grace.

> *Nanak says that God with His merciful look, showers happiness on them.*

This pauri concludes with Guru Nanak stating that the purpose of this human life is fulfilled when we receive the Divine Nectar, which brings us to wholeness and forever merges us into oneness with God.

The templates described above, continence, patience, understanding, daily practice, and devotion, are the tools to become the form of God in our own lives. These are the keys to a life of excellence and service—the keys to happiness.

The Form of God

The Guru is the form of God upon which we can meditate, imagine, and love. The practice of Kundalini Yoga enables us to embody the form of the Guru and to fulfill the words of the Guru. But how is this done? By developing our levers and lenses, our angles and triangles, we make of our limited human form a correct vehicle for the infinite *shakti* energy. Living our destiny requires energy; for that matter, so does living our fate. It takes less energy—physically, mentally, and emotionally—to live in the Guru's identity. With the Guru's guidance, we can be brought into a state of balance. A sense of ease, or *sahej*, is the fruit of this conscious way of living.

Just as our bodies show the wear and tear of living against the forces of nature, they also show the grace and ease of living in alignment with the forces of nature. What keeps us from making the better choice? Our ego's attachment to the familiar, the known, keeps us from making new choices. But this is where we can put our ego to good use—to change our form. The ego can be used to cultivate the disciplines of transformation, as well as to resist any influences to conform to distortion. Rather than continuing to allow the ego's projection to determine our lives, we can use the ego to move our lives in the direction we want.

How we move greatly influences our form. It begins with a thought, that thought becomes a feeling, and we breathe and move according to our feelings. Everything influences our thoughts and, in turn, our feelings: genetics, parents, environment, nature, nurture, even what we had for breakfast. We act under the influence of our feelings. These actions, these repeated movements within the field of gravity, create our form. We are influenced not only by Earth's gravitational field but also by the moon's, which creates the movement of the tides. The moon pulls on us, as do the sun and other planetary bodies. We are constantly being pushed and pulled into a form. We project that form out into the world, and the world responds in kind. Yet these influences are secondary to what lies at the core—the you in you being you. Yogi Bhajan reminded us so often to "just be you." But what does that mean? Hopefully, it means acting consciously, within the Guru's template, delivering your highest vibration—the You within you.

To fulfill our destiny, we must become aware of the influences that help or hinder our growth. Let's begin with looking at our food, medicines, vitamins, herbs, and supplements. It has been said that we are what we eat. The thirty trillion cells that make up our bodies vibrate the consciousness of the *prana*[33] they receive, the prana we give it: clean air, clean water, clean food. We may enjoy the taste of a salad. But once it's past the tongue, it delivers nutrients that nurture our cells to full radiant health. Building the body temple to serve our destinies requires knowing what we really need to fuel our lives. Making intelligent choices regarding the foods we consume, as well as medicines and herbal supplements, is a great first step. If the body is not well cared for nutritionally, the weaknesses that ensue distract us from our meditation and the fulfillment of our destiny. Yogi Bhajan recognized that food was both a nutritional and a spiritual supplement necessary for health and well being. If the foods we eat weaken our bodies, then our ability to move, breathe and think freely is compromised. The body organizes our perceptions of the world; food can create positive or negative associations in the mind, which affects our interactions in the world. Certain foods might cause us to become stiff and inflexible, comprising not only our ability to sit and meditate but also our ability to compromise in relationships. If the foods we eat irritate the connective tissues, then we might find ourselves being

33 The life force

irritable with our families or in our commute each morning. Foods can either support our values or compromise them. What we're willing to put into our bodies says a lot about how we value this body temple.

Another major influence on the foods we eat and their effect on the body temple is our attitude toward the food as we eat it. Being conscious of what we eat requires reverence. We influence our body's capacity to absorb the nutrients in the food, as well as the food's capacity to merge with us, by eating with an attitude of gratitude. Instead of taking food in, grasping for it in hunger, we receive it in gratitude. Many traditions offer prayers before eating that invoke God to "bless this food we are about to receive." After offering the food to God, we receive the blessing, through God's name, in both body and spirit.

In the Sikh tradition, a sweet food called Guru's *prasad*, a blessing, is served. It is made with sugar, flour, clarified butter, and water. At first glance, these ingredients might seem like the beginnings of a good dessert, not the source of spiritual and physical sustenance. But these ingredients are cooked and combined as a meditation; the one who prepares the prasad recites Guru Nanak's *Japji Sahib* throughout every step of the process: cooking the flour, butter, and sugar; pouring the water; and watching as the two liquids become one form. The vibration of God's word infuses the prasad; the prasad is then offered to the Guru, where it is further infused with devotional kirtan and the strength of a steel kirpan. At the end of the Sikh devotional service (Gurdwara), the prasad is served to the community (the *sangat*), who receive it with open hands and open hearts. This act of faith is processed by the body, delivering a blessing of the Guru's Grace to every cell. The sweetness anchors the memory of God's sweet love. The art of receiving a blessing is to experience *Ang Sang Wahe Guru.* With every cell and fiber of my body, God's Name is sung, trillions of cells dancing in the light of God's Name. The cells of this body temple serve the soul, continuously dying and being reborn, regenerating and changing with every new generation. As the forms of the cells change, they influence our overall form, our body temple.

I believe that in addition to the food we eat, how we breathe, or the quality of our breath, influences our body temple—and our spirit— more than anything else. The importance of breathing cannot be overemphasized. The cells of the body must be oxygenated. How we breathe influences how cells absorb oxygen. Shallow breathing is the biggest impediment to cellular oxygenation—specifically, insufficient exhalation. When we fail to expel enough of the old air, we recirculate the existing carbon dioxide in our lungs and effects the efficiency of the respitory system. This contributes to a great deal of stress and weakness throughout the body's various systems. From underoxygenated cells to changing the acid balance of the blood, how we breathe influences how we feel. Breathing mechanizes emotions; breathing in a shallow, anxious manner not only stresses muscles but also causes the brain to produce the fight-or-flight hormones adding to our stress. Whereas, a conscious exhale sets the foundation for an oxygen-sufficient inhale, decreasing our stress.

The Chakras

We've discussed the templates of the physical body and the habits that support it. Now let us explore the mystical anatomy of the human experience—the *chakras*, or energy centers. As the kundalini enters the different chakras, we experience the realities associated with them.

The First Chakra is associated with the earth element. Our basic relationship to Mother Earth is formed by the energies of this chakra where we feel nurtured and provided for. Any distortions of this chakra are primarily due to our mother phobias, which can greatly limit our ability to root and connect to the earth. The Root Chakra is also associated with the sense of smell. As things break down to their base elements, they smell bad. If our relationship to the root is out of balance, then our capacity to align is compromised. It is our inability to connect properly to the mother element that distorts that most basic alignment. The goal of yoga is to allow the kundalini to ascend to the Crown Chakra; but if the root is compromised, then the journey is misaligned from the start.

Learning how to sit and be connected to Mother Earth helps us become patient in our transformation. So often, we react compulsively, grasping and taking instead of waiting and receiving. As a result, our journey to higher consciousness usually fails. The First Chakra is typically blocked by fear—our basic fear that we will not be provided for, that our fundamental needs won't be met. If we believe that our basic needs are unmet, then we try to meet them ourselves. We take from the earth without gratitude. Our behavior becomes guided by fear, and our personalities become manipulative; our life's energy is spent getting our needs met. Those whose energies are blocked at the First Chakra become trapped in a "take or be taken" mentality. The fruit of this consciousness is selfishness, narcissism, and insecurity. If we live in this most fundamental form of fear, our actions and motivations become perverse. To succeed in removing fear related to the First Chakra from our lives, we require a remothering process.

Most people cannot sit on the floor with the spine straight because of difficulties with the First Chakra and the associated limitations of the hips and lower spine. Sitting up straight in the company of the Holy and singing divine hymns helps to heal the First Chakra; the security we long for is fulfilled by the grace of the Guru. Root Lock, or *mulbandh*, teaches us the most basic principal of the body—contract in order to expand. In addition, the tension from this lock puts pressure on the urogenital muscles, which develop strength and the purification required for our continued growth. For the *shushmana*, or energy channel, to constantly vibrate, the proper connection between the Root and Crown Chakras must be developed. The Crown Chakra, or Seventh Chakra, is the final connection between pure consciousness and Earth. When the kundalini pierces the Crown Chakra, oneness and connection with all is obtained, this state is known as *samadhi*. But this oneness is blocked by the ego. We cling to a limited identity and thus keep ourselves from our own experience of our true identity in infinity. Our attachment to ego, even the spiritual ego, limits our union.

The journey through the chakras is not direct. Instead, the chakras interact with one another through the subtle energetic channels, the *nadis*—the subtle and gross nerve channels that communicate to all parts of our being. These *nadis* flow along the spine and intersect at the seven chakras. There are two main *nadis*: the *ida* and *pingala*. Ida, begins on the left, is associated with the moon and brings cooling energies to the chakras. Pingala, on the right, brings the sun's energies—heat and vitality. These energies flow back and forth, moving through the seven chakras, culminating at the Crown Chakra.

The Guru says, "The Muladhara Chakra is pierced, and I have without doubt met the King. I have thus ended my attachment to Maya. The Moon has swallowed the Sun. When my breath was held to maximum filled capacity, the *Anaahad veen* resounds."[34]

34 *Siri Guru Granth Sahib*, page 972, Saint Kabir, 15th Century Sufi Saint

What does this poetic language speak of? The Root Chakra (the Muladhara) is pierced by the energy of the kundalini. The full moon, a symbol of the Crown Chakra, swallows the sun; the polarities of *ida* and *pingala*, soul and body, human and divine, have found resolution through the experience of the kundalini rising. And finally, when he experiences mastery over the prana, the breath, he hears the unstruck sound. For the *shushmana* to constantly vibrate the unstruck divine song, the proper connection between the first and seventh chakras must be developed.

The Guru says: "In the monastery of the six chakras, the detached mind resides. The power to listen to the sound vibrating within is awakened. The unstruck music plays, my mind is atuned to it. Through the Guru's word I am delighted by the True Name."[35]

So how do we unite the *nadis* and move from the root to the crown? The human body is formed from the basic elements of earth, water, fire, air, and ether, with each element corresponding to one of the first five chakras. I have already mentioned, in brief, the first and seventh centers; now let's introduce the other chakras. The Second Chakra represents the water element. Our emotions flow along with the hormones and fluids, influencing our feelings. We generate our feelings through our thinking and actions. The body is mostly made of water, and the circulation of these fluids affects our emotional life.

According to an ancient saying, "No pleasure should be taken." Animals can take what they need without consequence, but not humans. Nevertheless, we love to "take pleasure;" yet taking what is not given creates guilt. The Second Chakra's block is guilt. We suffer from guilty pleasures, with sex being the most prominent. Centered in the Second Chakra, sex is part of our most basic

---

35 *Siri Guru Granth Sahib*, page 907, Line 8, Guru Nanak Dev Ji

human instinct, as well as a large part of the creative process. We create ideas and bring new forms into our world; we even create life by giving birth. This creative aspect of the Second Chakra is a polarity to the Sixth Chakra, our intuition, which recognizes how to expand our creative expression into our world. If our sexual expression loses its sacredness, then we, in turn, lose the ability to access our deepest intuition; our feelings become distorted, and our actions betray our divine nature. We remain animalistic. We lose our subtlety and our intuition is compromised.

In order to gain our "angel eyes," we must conquer our inner beast and learn to bless what we receive. When we enjoy the fruits of our intuition along with the fruits of the world—food, sex, art, among many others—we remove our inner duality. When we increase our appreciation, guilt subsides. Guilt often acts as a warning. When we begin to feel guilty about the actions or thoughts we have taken, it is essentially a feeling that prevents the kundalini from bringing proper understanding to the Second Chakra. This guilt also disrupts the Sixth Chakra, because as our feelings grow distorted, so too does our intuition. The Sixth Chakra's primary block is duality. Our water-based feelings cause us to experience life as a series of dualities—good against bad, black against white, up against down—which creates separation instead of unity. Part of healing the Second and Sixth chakras requires practicing oneness with ourselves. We must develop a one-pointed mind and control over the movement of the water element. The quickest way to become one-pointed is through the eyes by developing a *dhristi*—holding the eyes at fixed points, such as the Third Eye or the tip of the nose, brings things into oneness. The water element is controlled by applying *mulbandh*. If done with proper devotion and self-forgiveness, correct contraction at the first three centers, along with the eyes held steady, can help heal us from guilt and its inherent duality.

The Third Chakra is the fire element and is in polarity to the Fifth Chakra, and the ether element. Located at the navel, its domain is fire, heat, and light. The first three chakras make up what is known as the lower triangle. This is the chalice of our feminine nature, which supplies and supports the heart center. We have already discussed the Navel Point's vital role in developing our physical wisdom. As kundalini energy pierces the Navel Point and the *nadis* merge in the *shushmana*, the profound power of the *prana* is made available. But this power can be blocked by feeling ashamed. On the other hand, the heat of the navel can bring energy to the darker sides of the ego: anger, lust, greed, pride, and attachment. These traditional vices are all fed by lower triangle energies. If guilt doesn't cause us to rethink and heal our behavior, then comes the infamous pride before the fall. Humiliation causes an emotional and physical collapse. Our posture weakens as the heart weighs more heavily on the navel. As the heart collapses, the facial muscles are drawn down as well. This blocks the kundalini.

The fire element is what puts the heat into emotions, especially anger. Anger can only be healed with forgiveness. To allow the shame to heal, we must learn to forgive ourselves and give ourselves permission to receive God's love. This transmutes the heat of anger into strength and support for the heart center, bringing the ensuing light. The navel supports the diaphragm which moves the air, and gives us our voice. Shame, which compromises the navel, also alters our speech. The kundalini cannot move freely through the Throat Chakra because the lower body's distortion also distorts the neck and head. The Throat Chakra is the sound chakra; its highest characteristic is speaking truth. This chakra is most commonly blocked by lies, especially the lies we tell ourselves. When we speak from fear and anger, we try to buy time with our lies, but instead we block ourselves from the truth. We become our words. Either we can expand in the form of God and Guru, or we can contract in the form of our fears, angers, and despair. When the Third Chakra is in dynamic relationship to the Fifth Chakra, the navel supports our words and our words expand our identity, rooted in the fire of the navel. The relationship is symbiotic and supportive of our infinite identity in truth.

The Heart Chakra rules the experience of being human. Receiving from the chakras above and below, its element is air, where the breath—the "holy spirit"—brings the elements into form. Love and its virtues emanate from the Heart Chakra. When the Heart Chakra is open and purified, one sees the Lord in the heart and is imbued, in every cell, by the Lord. This is the experience of the *amrit*, the holy nectar. The blocks of this chakra are many, but unique to each of us, and can include feeling disconnected from our soul, grief, broken-hearted, shadow-hearted, loneliness, lack of self-love, jealousy and insecurity. With the kundalini awakened and its ascent complete, the divine nectar trickles down to bring the essence of the immortal. When the heart is awakened, the kundalini can freely ascend and descend through the Seven Chakras. This state of realization concludes with the kundalini piercing the Crown Chakra. The lotus flower then opens, creating a crown of divinity, protection, and grace. Through the Heart Chakra, we experience how the basic elements come to life with the seed from above and the vitality from below, all born from the spirit and breath of love.

Three Things Worth Learning: Sit, Stand, and Walk

 Sit

Learning to sit allows us to be comfortable in our bodies and get to know ourselves, as well as enjoy a deeper relationship with the Guru. I became aware of the importance of sitting well, along with the challenges that come from sitting on the floor, at a young age. When I was seven years old, I belonged to a YMCA organization known as Indian Guides. This father-son activity group focused on learning the ways of the Native American culture, and a large part of our activities involved learning about nature, including camping, hiking, tracking, hunting, and fishing. But more than the activities, it was about father-son bonding and the opportunity for a father's wisdom to be shared. We would sit in a circle for the wisdom council, "Indian style," and pass around the talking stick when we had a question or something to share. I remember my father not enjoying the council meetings because of his inability to sit comfortably on the ground—and he wasn't the only one. As children, we sat straight quite comfortably, but most of our fathers were slumped over and uncomfortable. We would meet weekly and practice our version of Native American wisdom, with the deeper purpose of this practice being to connect and commune with the feminine—our Mother Earth. I enjoyed sitting on the ground and feeling a direct connection to the earth. Certain Native tribes of the American Plains believed that Mother Earth spoke to their hearts through the sit bones at the base of the pelvis. They learned to sit and listen to their Mother Earth as she spoke about the weather, the buffalo migration, and the location of any enemies. In most cultures, humans start their lives sitting on the floor as children and but then move to desks as they grew older. I am personally not against desks, but I am absolutely for maintaining a lifelong ability to comfortably sit on the floor.

Breath and Bones

The Throne of the Heart

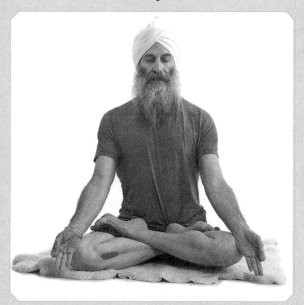

This is a visualization I often practice, even for just a few minutes. I sit on the floor, sit bones properly connected to the earth. Establishing good alignment allows better concentration because the meditation is not disturbed by physical discomfort. In this seat, I become a throne of consciousness. On this throne, in the center of my heart, sits my Guru, the Raj Yogi; and in His presence I gaze into my own inner kingdom. I experience the body as a throne for the Guru's presence. The outer throne is the physical body and the inner throne is the heart center. The heart center is a lotus throne made into a seat of virtues. On this seat of virtues sits my Guru. The virtues and the comforts of alignment make for an inviting place to sit. This is really a personal assessment of my own effort to become better through truthful living.

In Gurdwara, I sit for the blessing of the whole community in the presence of the Guru. To be able to sit straight in the presence of the Guru is a blessing, whether in someone's home or at the Golden Temple in Amritsar, it's an experience of our own majesty. Sitting correctly brings calmness. Better posture also frees the muscles that support the thoracic diaphragm, which allows the voice to more comfortably participate in the joyful noise of devotional singing.

The great challenge of sitting comfortably results from the distortion of our postures. We can't sit up straight because of structural weaknesses of the muscles and nerves. The body begins to age at the sacrum, the fused bone at the base of the spine. Sacrum means "sacred" or "to sacrifice." The muscles of the navel and those that line the inner bowl of the pelvis and connect to the sacrum need to be used in an intelligently applied sacrifice in order to try and create balance and alignment in the pelvis. The Navel and the uro-genital muscles are often the first to weaken because of basic, structural misalignment issues in the pelvis and overall. The pelvic alignment is also influenced by emotional and sexual issues, which cause further alignment difficulties. Retraining these muscle groups is necessary to heal and improve alignment. We learn the basic science of Mulbandh by contracting these muscles to expand through the chest while also better connecting to the earth through the sit bones.

The muscles of the pelvic floor serve many functions. One of the least understood of these functions is how these muscles are used to connect the sit bones to the floor. This downward connection, grounding or rooting, creates an upward lift, which directly supports the heart and head. Because we have not been properly trained to root down in order to rise up, our alignment often becomes distorted. A common misconception about core strength is that abdominal strength is the essence of core strength. This understanding is misleading because it's incomplete. A trinity makes us core conscious. This trinity begins with the core values, which are our heart's virtues. How we hold our heart reflects what we hold in our hearts. How we carry the container of these virtues reflects our relationship to what is in the container. The science of how we carry our hearts is our body's core intelligence. This is the basis for the angles and triangles of Kundalini Yoga. All asanas and postures, when done correctly, maintain a correct relationship to the heart center. The repetitive relationship between core intelligence and

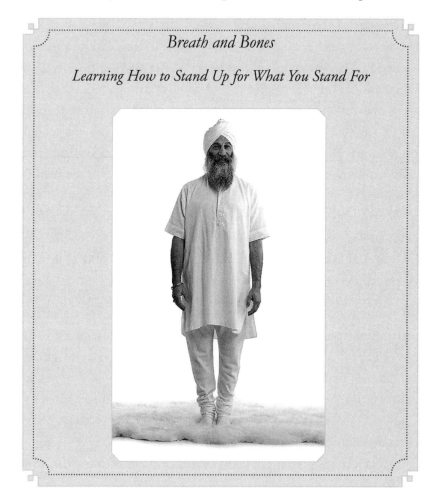

Breath and Bones

Learning How to Stand Up for What You Stand For

core values gives core stregth. This, in turn, inspires our maxim: Obey, serve, love, and excel in the service of the Heart Master. We express what we experience. Everything moves to and from the heart. Our body language and facial expressions show the outer world our own inner world. Our emotions live on our faces, dwell in our bodies, and affect our breath patterns.

Knowing the science of how to correctly stand is an important part of a yogic education. A good place to begin this discussion is at the Navel Point. The classic Navel Point is, depending on a person's size, about one to two inches below the belly button. When we engage the Navel Point, we bring balance, grace, and smoothness to the way we bend, bow, stand, walk, jump, punch, sing, speak, and even laugh. The properly educated navel can effectively communicate not only alignment and posture patterns but also speech. A properly educated navel means knowing how to apply the mulbandh, correctly contracting the muscles of the navel, sex organ, and anus. The navel orchestrates a correct relationship with the pelvis, energetically lengthening downward through the legs and allowing the feet to better connect to the earth. The feet, when aligned properly from the core, spread the four corners of each foot into the earth. Properly aligned from the navel point, the twenty-six bones in each foot can be used for better balance. From the grounding of the feet, the base of our stance is established. The properly aligned pelvis becomes our foundation. With this foundation and our hearts resting in the proper place, the head can float on the shoulders and see the path ahead with clarity and freedom. In my stance, I try to be powerful at the navel, smooth with the breath through the chest, and subtle in lengthening my neck and head.[1]

1   See *Divine Alignment* by Guru Prem Singh Khalsa for more information on the bandhas and the breath.

Stand

Sometimes I ask myself, "What do I stand for? Do I stand on principle? Will I have the courage to take a stand when time and space require it? Can I stand my ground? Or will I complain that I can't stand it?" Each morning, I sing the *Song of the Khalsa*, which has the line, "Stand as the Khalsa, strong as steel, steady as stone, give our lives to God and Guru, mind and soul, breath and bone."[36] This is the essence of what I stand for. This idea is strongly influenced by our beliefs, as well as our skill at balancing our emotions and feelings through the muscles, bones, and nerves. To become a stand-up person, it is important to learn the science of standing. If we're to stand for righteousness, we must know how to hold onto our inner virtues. If we don't want to be shaky or weak in the knees, we require guidance on the science of standing and training with proper posture. What we hold in our hearts affects how we hold our hearts. If we value our own virtues, then we will be valued for what we stand for and how we stand by other people. If you live your life on a proper "footing," you will be able to "foot" the bill and say, "My pleasure."

Even when we are just standing around, there is a dynamic dance happening in, around and through us. We are never really just standing still. Maintaining a proper standing alignment requires constant, yet subtle, adjustments. We have all been told at least once to stand up straight. But standing up straight is more about a balancing act than a "holding" act. Remember, root down, rise up, then release any unnecessary tension. With these skills, we can be like a tree firmly rooted but able to sway with the wind, yielding and growing. Otherwise with branches too stiff and roots too weak, we cannot stand the test of time. In the end, we all want to be grounded in our principles and face steadily whatever comes our way.

36 "Song of the Khalsa" written by Livtar Singh Khalsa

Breath and Bones

Tall as a Tree

Practicing Tree Pose is a good example of what a rooted connection to the earth looks like. When done properly, the Tree Pose allows us to experience a root line into the earth through each foot. This root line is established at the navel and organically and energetically connects the body to the earth at the point of contact. When standing on the feet, the connection is from the Navel Point to the feet. When doing a handstand, the connection is from the Navel Point to the hands. The navel supports the heart to receive the energies and wisdom that flow from the root. In the case of tree pose, one foot is firmly planted on the earth, balance as you lift your other foot and bring the heel as high as you can toward your groin with the sole of the foot pressing into the thigh of the standing leg. Focus on something stationary, and use your core to grow roots energetically from the navel, through your standing leg; feel your kneecap lift. Practice being a firmly rooted tree.

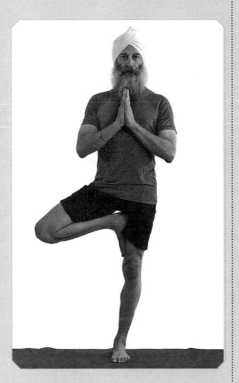

Walk

"There was a crooked man, and he walked a crooked mile"—this line from a children's nursery rhyme sums up the way in which many people move through life. The crooked man has no idea he isn't moving straight; that is just the state of his world. Most people move through life not knowing where they are going. The journey toward our destinies defines our lives. What would a man of God walk like? In Yogi Bhajan's poem "The Calling," he says, "In the walk of life, in the dance of life, we all kiss the pranic breath. In the total surroundings of our wonderful world we are born to find our depth. We have to walk on the path of the self, to find our own grace."

My father had a distinct walk. With a heavy heel, his sound was distinct, and I could always tell when he was home even without seeing him. I inherited my father's walk. This wasn't a genetic inheritance but an energetic one. I had subconsciously copied his walking pattern. I walked with my feet turned out and my heels hitting heavily with each step. But this way of walking weakens the spine and tightens the hips. The way we walk both reflects and affects who we are and where we are going. After listening to Yogi Bhajan talk about "walking on our paws," I made a great effort to change my walk. According to Yogi Bhajan, we need to properly use the balls of our feet in order to walk smoothly and quietly. Walking with a gentle spring in the step has been shown to increase vitality and even longevity, even shoe manufacturers have caught on. Changing the way we walk is a bit like changing the way we talk. It takes committed practice to change and improve something we've done so many times. I began to realize that when I walked with my feet turned out, I felt life coming at me like a head wind. Although walking with my feet parallel took practice, it now feels like I'm cutting through space and time more effectively and smoothly.

A major part of my personal transformation has involved healing my inner anger. Yogi Bhajan referred to my variety of inner anger as "professional anger." I was angry that God wasn't doing a better job, according to me. To heal my professional anger, I needed to be able to bless all and fix a few. One of the ways I practice blessing all is while I'm walking. I imagine myself as a blessing machine. Whatever light might be in me I project to everybody; good, bad, broken, beautiful—everyone gets blessed. I attempt to touch all with my inner light. I want my breath connected to my inner light so that it expands and touches all; it's a universal embrace through the breath. My ego doesn't do the blessing, nor do I want any recognition for any light that might come from somewhere within me. As a Sikh, I don't proselytize, but I do advertise. And what do I advertise? My spirit, character, posture, dignity, divinity, and grace—I try to put all of these into my smile and take them out for a walk.

Breath and Bones

Walking Meditation

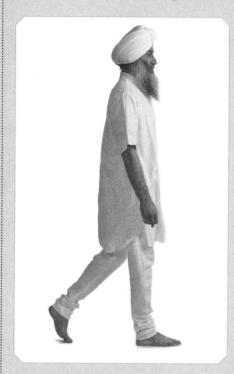

My favorite walking meditation is to listen to Jaap Sahib while walking.[37] I enjoy walking to the rhythm of this bani. Sometimes I do various breath walks while listening to Jaap Sahib or the sound of the inner mantra. My favorite breath walk is to coordinate the Breath of Fire while walking. To do this walking pranayama, you must be well practiced at doing Breath of Fire correctly. Begin by walking correctly: Exhale and engage the navel as the ball of your foot presses to the ground and then inhale as the foot lifts up. With each foot engagement, exhale pushing and inhale lifting up. It may take some practice to become smooth and coordinated. You can build this breath walk up to 11 minutes. I believe this walking pranayama is one of the most powerful cardiovascular exercises a human can do.

---

37 Please note: Yogi Bhajan taught *charan jaap*, walking meditation; this is the author's personal interpretation of these practices.

Walking Tall

Another example of walking consciously was on the 1970s' TV show *Kung Fu*. Cain, the protagonist and budding Kung Fu Master, was told that when he could successfully walk across the floor without tearing the delicate rice paper covering, then he would be able to walk without being heard. Tread lightly—that is, walk through life quietly, leaving behind no noise, no footprints, and no monuments to the ego. My goal is to walk this path, becoming my name each step of the way.

In my younger days, I used to slump as I walked, with my feet turned out and my heels hitting hard. But now I practice walking consciously. I make a greater effort to walk tall and to be light on my feet. I carry my "hearts" as the valuable gifts they are, because my virtues are what I value most. I don't try to hold my head up high; instead, I balance it as a level head on my shoulders. While my level head navigates my safe journey, my wise heart rules and leads the way, and my intelligent navel orchestrates and distributes the energies to get me where I'm going. While walking, I roll off the balls of my feet to put a bit of a spring into my step, and I allow my arms to swing freely with each step. This is the outer aspect of walking. But another, inner aspect of walking well is to move as an example of a happy person. If you walk happily, you bring hope to the neighborhood. It is also important for me to walk with a smile. For years, I had to fake a smile before it became natural to my face. Now I often push my tongue to the upper pallet of my mouth to make my smiling more of a meditation. Walking with happiness is a lifetime meditation, and I encourage everyone to become a lighthouse of joy and peace that blesses all.

My father once told me, "Son, the most important thing you will ever learn, in what I hope is a long life, is when it is time to die." What he meant was to not extend your own life at the expense of another innocent human being. Because of our heritage, the example he used was from the Nazi concentration camps. Sometimes prisoners were allowed to live if they assisted the Nazis with the deaths of their fellow prisoners. He said, "If the time ever comes when you must choose between saving your own life at the cost of another's, death is the right choice." Although my father never sang the *Song of the Khalsa*, he was essentially sharing with me the first line of that song: "Many speak of courage, speaking cannot give it; it's in the face of death that we must live it." With Guru-guided courage, we can always know in our hearts where we stand and which path we will walk. Yogi Bhajan taught that if we walk on the path of destiny, destiny runs toward us. If we know where we're going, small steps can turn for us a very big wheel .

The heart is the hub of all sacred places; go there and roam.
—Anonymous

Chapter Five

Kundalini Awakening

*The Sikh who follows the path of devotion meditates on the Naam,
Har Har Har Har. Fixing his mind in the breath, at the navel point,
energy turns round and round up the shushmana, as it opens, vibrating,
consciousness rises, the thousand-petal lotus blooms, nectar trickles
down, such a being merges with Brahm.*

—Yogi Bhajan, in Furmaan Khalsa

Kundalini—the first time I heard this word was in high school.
The year was 1971, and I was in the eleventh grade. My high
school was the first, anywhere, to offer Kundalini Yoga. A few of
my closest friends were taking the class and encouraged me to
participate. I remember my best friend asking me, "Don't you
want to experience the kundalini?" He proclaimed that it would be

better than anything I had ever experienced. Up to that point, my experience with yoga had been limited to looking at Sivananda's *Complete Illustrated Book of Yoga* and trying some of the postures. As a gymnast, the stretches seemed useful but not really necessary for me.

My first book of wisdom was Baba Ram Dass' *Be Here Now*. Maybe it was the way it was presented, or maybe it was me, but his words connected with me, and I was beginning to awaken. My teenage emotions and feelings were being confronted by a consciousness that jumped off the pages of this groundbreaking book. During this same period, I also read Herman Hess' *Siddartha*. I related to the insulated and protected world in which Prince Siddartha lived. But I doubted that I could ever leave my "comfortable" life.

I identified with the hippie movement but was too young to fully participate. I was living through one of the greatest shifts in human consciousness. The counterculture was in full swing, and it showed up everywhere: music, clothes, language, and politics. *Kundalini* was just another word from the expanding vocabulary of the "hippie" movement. Yoga was part of the new awareness that included many other Indian philosophical traditions. It was a time of incense, paisley shirts, Ravi Shankar, transcendental meditation, and a host of other new cultural icons and ideas. All of this was further energized by the Vietnam War, which presented me with the very real possibility of being drafted into the army. Something desperately wanted to wake up from within me. The signs were everywhere, even the word *kundalini* itself sounded so familiar and yet so mysterious.

This was not my first introduction to the powers within. Even before I was going to Indian Guides with my father, I would sit under a densely shaded tree in my backyard and imagine being part of a small herd of buffalo. This activity was greater than imagination for me; I truly experienced a connection. The buffalo were like my guardian spirits, and I often practiced this buffalo "meditation" in order to return to that space in which I felt both peace and great power. I know now that this was a state of expanded consciousness—a kundalini awakening. My backyard peace competed with the challenges and pressures of growing up in the 1950s and 1960s. There was no other place in my life for this type of consciousness. My parents tolerated my buffalo fantasies and even found them amusing, but what they really wanted was for me to excel. They pushed me to excel in the outer world; so I gave up inner peace for outer recognition.

So, there I was, in high school, able to command the attention of my peers (and girls—don't forget the attention of girls) because of my skills with gymnastics and music; yet all the while I was being confronted from within. I knew that my motivation was all wrong. I was being offered the opportunity to reconnect with what my heart and soul really wanted, but I couldn't let go of my ego's need for recognition. Honestly speaking, a large part of my motivations was like so many of my generation: Work hard to be recognized and get high to ease the loneliness.

My friends, who were instrumental in getting me to try so many other hippie methods of altering my consciousness, such as smoking and drinking, were now influencing me to try Kundalini Yoga; so I joined in and began being instructed in a new way of breathing, thinking, and moving. I was learning about mantras. I listened, tried the exercises, did the breathing, chanted the mantras, but had little commitment to or investment in this new way of life. Although I was very curious, I was equally insecure; so I told my friends that I was a gymnast and therefore didn't need yoga.

In all honesty, however, I knew right away that yoga was exactly what I needed, but I was unwilling to give up my false comforts. My Kundalini Yoga friends had given up drugs, alcohol, and meat, and they wanted me to join them. But I just wanted us to continue in our old way of life. So we grew apart. I continued my gymnastics, and they continued their yoga practice.

I knew from prior experiences that there was a great power hiding itself within me. I was often reminded of that power when it would reappear. Sometimes, while flipping, flying, and balancing, I would feel this incredible energy moving through me, making the impossible seem easy. It was a tease, though, because it was unsustainable; but God had given me a taste of what was possible, without causing irreparable damage.

During my Christmas break in 1971, while attending a gymnastics camp, I first met Dan Millman. At that time, he was the gymnastics coach at Stanford University. It would be another nine years before his classic book, *Way of the Peaceful Warrior*, would be published. But his workshops were my first exposure to Eastern principals as they applied to gymnastics. Dan talked about the navel and developing the Ki energy, which could be harnessed for creative expression. He taught that doing less brought more. At 17, I believed that the ego needed to be strengthened not relaxed. Yet Dan explained that explosive power requires relaxation and calm. Although I was really drawn to his ideas, I didn't have a way to incorporate them into my life and practice. I knew that the Ki energy needed to be cultivated to allow an awakening of my true potential, but it would take another four years before I would take my first "real" Kundalini Yoga class. The seed, however, had been planted, again.

Another experience that coincided in my 17th year was my parents insisting that I experience rolfing, also known as structural integration. Through a specific type of deep tissue massage, tensions are released and posture is improved. Rolfer's theorize that the body holds deep emotional patterns in the muscles and connective tissues. Rolfing techniques hope to free the body-mind of these emotional limitations. My own experience with rolfing was remarkable. It helped free my body from certain limitations and more quickly expand my gymnastic expertise. It was around this time that I began to realize that I was only using a small part of my potential. I began to focus on improving my posture as a continuous meditation. My gymnastic alignment improved, as did the way I stood and walked.

In addition to rolfing, I was introduced to the Alexander system, which focuses on technical alignment of the body through selective movement patterns. I studied this system for two years, refining my body's relationship to gravity. In addition, I spent time studying several other modalities, including the Feldenkrais method. All of these bodywork modalities added to my experience of awareness through movement.

From age 17 to 22, I lived in great duality. I was equally drawn to the forces of dark and light. I had always had an inner guide, but I also had a lot of inner pain. I dealt with the pain by going to "sleep" for four years. In college, I distanced myself from the possibility of transformation and rejected the counterculture. I adopted the philosophy and lifestyle of a politically conservative elitist, a person of privilege. I joined a fraternity and convinced myself that that was where my future lay. Having a career and making money were all that mattered. I fabricated a persona that was both fact and fiction, but entirely untrue to my soul. I knew I needed to wake up, the signs were everywhere, but I couldn't let go of the darkness. I battled with the devil and the divine from high school through college, occasionally remembering that this was not the life I came to live. The buffalo haunted me.

The one place where the counterculture continued to have its sway over me was music. In the early 1970s, I was drawn to music that spoke of the lowest and highest aspects of the human spirit. The Beatles—especially George Harrison—offered insights into what was best and worst in our human potential. The warnings and the guidance were there in the words and melodies. From *Beware of Darkness* to *My Sweet Lord*, George was offering what seemed to me at the time to be a personal invitation to wake up. Pete Townsend of The Who brought the life of devotion into the then secular world of sex, drugs, and rock and roll. The album *Who's Next* played out like an anthem of devotion. When Pete became a devotee of Meher Baba, it was the most creative period of his life. When I listened to songs like *Bargain* and *Parvatigar*, they reminded me of a place I hadn't visited in a long time. I would sing along with the music and experience, once again, the presence of my soul begging to be recognized. But I still wasn't ready to receive the gift.

Movies also conspired to wake me up. Bruce Lee's *Enter the Dragon* provided evidence of the hidden power that could be harnessed, once awakened. I too wanted to find this power and realize my creative potential. My kundalini was awakening, but the pattern of its assent wasn't steady, and it was often sabotaged by my impulsive and emotional behavior. I wasn't fully committed to the process. I needed a teacher. Looking back, I see that Yogi Bhajan's poem "Wake Up," in *Furmaan Khalsa*, described my struggle perfectly. How serendipitous it is that he eventually became my teacher.

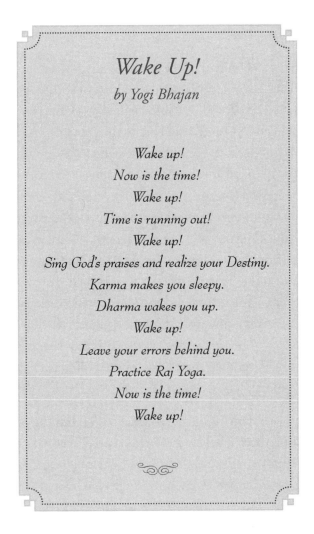

Wake Up!
by Yogi Bhajan

Wake up!
Now is the time!
Wake up!
Time is running out!
Wake up!
Sing God's praises and realize your Destiny.
Karma makes you sleepy.
Dharma wakes you up.
Wake up!
Leave your errors behind you.
Practice Raj Yoga.
Now is the time!
Wake up!

One of the greatest benefits from all my somatic and gymnastic training was that the training put into stark contrast the difference between my physical experience and my spiritual reality. The lightness of my body contradicted the darkness in my soul. Although my outer body was well fed, my soul was starving. I knew what I needed: a committed life of meditation, prayer, and service. The big question was who's prayer, meditation, and service?

Finding My Path

I was born into a family that was traditionally Jewish but religiously agnostic. They had very little use for religion or spirituality. I, on the other hand, suffered without spiritual food; so I began searching. I read, took classes, and searched within my own soul for my soul's food. I even attempted Orthodox Judaism. I went to various churches and looked into the Hari Krishna movement, because, after all, George Harrison was into it. At 22, as a senior at the University of Southern California, I began my study of pantomime and Kundalini Yoga. With these practices, I began to wake up. But it wasn't only me who was seeking and finding—others were beginning to wake up in their own way as well. It was interesting how many people I knew who were practicing different spiritual disciplines. Among my friends were Buddhists, Sufis, Hindus, Sikhs, Taoists, Christians, and Jews. I loved the commitment people brought to their practices, but I still wasn't clear which would become my chosen path.

For about a year, I ate from the spiritual buffet, but I kept returning to Kundalini Yoga, I believed it held a secret that was being held from me that I simply needed to find. At one point I was being counseled by a "super" Kundalini Yogi who would do the most difficult kriyas and meditations. I was in awe. He told me that if I intended to practice at the highest level of intensity, I would need a close, personal relationship with the Guru. Only 28 himself, he was doing the most difficult yoga practices under the guidance of Yogi Bhajan and had been instructed to read from the *Siri Guru Granth Sahib* every day to contain and guide the energy. At the time I asked myself, How could words of wisdom contain and guide the *pranic* force of the kundalini? And why these words and not some other?

Once I accepted the Guru, it seemed that I had been preparing my entire life to live as a Sikh, because I had always defined myself by my discipline. So, I moved into a Sikh ashram and began a brand new life. I had only planned on living in the ashram for a few months, and then I would return to my apartment and my "normal" life. I moved in and faced the challenge of getting up each day at 3:30 in the morning, practicing yoga, meditating, serving, and working in a community business that paid very little. I lived in a small house with 15 other people. I was challenged by the new lifestyle, but for the first time, my soul felt truly fed. The creative pressures of ashram living were perfect for accelerating my growth. I had never been asked to live for others, much less to share what I earned with others. This was the beginning of living as *we* instead of *me*. And from that we, I began to experience Thee. God consciousness was emerging from group consciousness. Thirty-four years later, and I am still living the ashram life, if in a slightly different form.

Soon after I moved into the ashram, when I was 23 years old, I had a remarkable experience. At the time, I was doing an average of two yoga sets a day, plus morning *sadhana*. Yet I still approached Kundalini Yoga like a gymnast; I wanted to conquer postures and kriyas. One day, I was doing the Navel Intelligence Kriya. One of the asanas is called *Raja Bhujangasana*, or King Cobra, a deep backbend in which you attempt to bring the feet up and over to touch the head from the standard Cobra Pose. I could always get close, but my feet never touched my head. However, on this one occasion, something different occurred. After doing the posture and nearly touching, I lowered down to the floor to relax; but rather than relaxing, I came back into the posture, and this time my spine opened and became quite hot. I then melted into the posture with my feet resting on my head. Moments later, a very powerful energy moved out of my lower spine and surged throughout my body and my being. I lost all sense of form. I stopped being a body and became energy. I had no dimension; instead, I was vibrating. I became filled with fear and felt trapped in a state of what seemed like perpetual fear. I recognized time but not space. I thought that I might remain there forever. I prayed to God to save me from this horrible fate. And then it happened—the vibration of fear became the vibration of love, and I began to reform. I returned to my human form and found myself lying on the floor completely soaked in sweat. What I had experienced was a transcendental state of fear. From that moment forward, my sense of reality was forever altered.

I wish I could say that I was transformed into a saint by that experience, but I wasn't. However, I did become more respectful of the powers within, and I increased my efforts to self realize. What the experience did was teach me to trust the God within me. It also moved me closer to my relationship to the True Guru, which continues to guide my life.

The Kundalini

The symbol of the kundalini is the cobra. Snakes are cold-blooded animals; they need the heat of the day to wake up. So, too, the sleeping human potential is symbolized by a coiled snake hibernating at the base of the spine. With properly applied heat, or *tapas*, the snake awakens from its slumber and begins to uncoil and rise.

Typically, when an animal awakens from hibernation, the first thing it wants to do is eat. Likewise, the kundalini eats up the darkness and illusions that separate humans from their true identity. Through the movement of the kundalini, the chakras are balanced and ultimately healed. The soul's light brightens as the chakras are cleansed of their karmas. Although the light of God is infused in every cell, God-consciousness comes once we've transcended the elements. When we put forth an effort to cleanse our bodies and our consciousness, the kundalini can rise and stimulate the heavenly nectar to drip down ultimately removing the sense of separation and merge us into unisoness with God.

The *nadis*—those 72,000 energy pathways—connect throughout the body-mind. The Guru says, "I have locked My breath at *Ida, Pingala*, and *Shushmana*. I have united the moon and the sun (Ida and pingala). The True Guru made the nectar juice flow. This has taken place in my tenth gate. There the unstruck melody plays, and in the sound of the word, I have spontaneously merged into a state of balance." Prana and apana, when mixed at the navel point, go down to enter the *Shushmana*, or central spinal energy channel, giving a charge to the Kundalini Shakti, which rises up this central channel and opens the chakras on its way to the tenth gate. This describes the rising of the kundalini into the light of God.

We have within us something that operates similar to superstring theory. When the body-mind is in balance, the *shushmana* awakens, and the divine music vibrates the central channel with God's song. In the world of Physics, superstring theorists believe, very simply stated, that the universes' multiple dimensions are composed of vibrating "strings". When we tune our mind and bodies to God's song, we become the vibrating instrument of God. There are many ways to approach the realization and cultivation of inner virtues. The Guru lays out a formula for success. However, it should be noted that partial success is often confused with true realization. Out-of-body experiences, or deep experiences within the body, can give a taste of the Lord's light. But if they become part of a spiritual ego, then the destiny is not fulfilled. I have had a few of these powerful but limited experiences, and I've learned a lot from them; but more important, I've learned they aren't the goal.

Kundalini Rising:
Tales of the Ordinary and the Extraordinary

The kundalini awakening can occur in many different ways. While flying combat missions in the Pacific Theater during World War II, my own father had experiences that resonate with the kundalini experience. As a child, I would ask him how he could have faced death on so many occasions. He told me something that I wouldn't understand until much later in my life. He described his combat missions to me in this way: At the start of the missions, he would be very focused on doing his job. But as they flew over the bombsites and the danger peaked, he described a calm stillness coming over him in that moment. He said it felt surreal—such calm in the face of death all around him.

This state of one-pointedness I have yet to achieve—that is, to face death fearlessly, calmly, and totally present. My father achieved a temporary state of no past or future, only the present moment. He said that he only experienced fear after the mission was complete, when he would think back on what had happened. Acting courageously while in the face of fear is one recognizable trait of the kundalini awakening. Throughout my childhood, I felt unable to face death like my father had. This capacity of his had influenced the rest of his life and had given him the courage to do many other things that he might not otherwise have tried.

Beyond courage, the affirmation, "Obey, Serve, Love, and Excel," also describes the kundalini awakening experience. Using my father's example again, his military training had taught him to obey and serve. That commitment allowed him to do his duty and face death. Death and love are difficult to reconcile. If his goal was to serve and possibly die, then the kundalini moved him enough. My father died when I was 23 years old, and though he suffered a difficult and painful disease at the end, I never saw him show any fear of death. He remained courageous until the end.

Until then, I had lived much of my life in fear. But after being witness to my father's life—and death—I became committed to finding courage. Not long after my father's death, I felt the freedom to live a very different life. And that's when the dharma entered the picture. In addition to living in an ashram, I began dressing in the traditional style of the Khalsa Sikh and began wearing a turban. The real tests of my commitment were about to begin. My family was very upset by the changes I was making, and we grew distant for some time. I had been working for my mother, assisting her in the field of neurokinesiology. But my new look and her worldview were a poor fit. It was time for me to seek employment elsewhere; so I became a gymnastics coach.

I believe I was the first turban-wearing gymnastics coach anywhere, or at least anywhere in the United States. I began coaching at my old high school, where I was reunited with my former high school coach. That was the first time I saw how powerful Kundalini Yoga could be in a purely athletic environment. Although I coached the team in the usual way in the afternoon, I requested that they also come to morning "conditioning," which was a Kundalini Yoga practice. Five days a week, we did kriyas and meditations. That season, the team became the best boys high school gymnastics team in the country. It is rare to see transformation happen so overtly. And it was more than athletic—many excelled in school and citizenship as well. The synergy of individuals becoming a group with a common purpose kept us in an exalted state of excellence.

I witnessed the collective team consciousness awaken and excel. What I discovered from my coaching experience was that my students were willing to explore and commit to new things because they trusted me. They trusted my skill, but they also trusted my discipline—I walked the talk.

I'd like to share one more story of the Kundalini awakening experience. In 1981, I was serving as a guide on an overnight camping trip. The trip was for 7- to 11-year old children during the annual Summer Solstice Celebrations. We were going to camp at Abiquiu Lake in northern New Mexico. Upon arriving at our campsite, we were all very hot and wanted to cool off in the lake. It was my decision to allow the children to go swimming, because I believed it would be safe for the kids to wade close to shore. As it turned out, it wasn't. While I was discussing the safety of the situation with another guide, a child's water buddy was sitting on the shore crying. This was our only clue that something had gone terribly wrong. The young girl said she couldn't find her swimming buddy. I immediately knew we had an emergency on our hands.

There was a child out there in the lake, and we didn't have a very clear idea where she might be. I entered the lake with another guide and started walking through the water. The water was muddy brown with little visibility. Only two of us were looking for our needle in this great haystack. The other guide was maybe 15 feet in front of me, slowly moving through 3 to 4 feet of water. As I watched him move in front of me, I had the sense that he knew where he was going. He would later claim that he had no idea. Yet I had felt a presence guiding him, and I felt this presence in me as well.

By now the child had been under water for over five minutes. Still, I felt this presence. Then the guide in front of me stopped, bent down, and picked up a young girl out of the muddy water. It was clear from the girl's appearance that she was dead. I had recently completed a CPR course, which was fortunate because I was the only one there with the necessary training. I took the girl, who was 8 years old, and laid her on the rocky shore. I became aware that there were 60 children looking on in shock at their dead friend. One of the other guides had the children form a circle around me and start chanting to Guru Ram Das. What happened next is difficult to describe clearly. I recall feeling calm but focused as I started the CPR, which included dislodging her tongue and starting her heart. I began to administer mouth-to-mouth resuscitation when I heard and experienced something miraculous. The children were chanting with so much devotion that they became one voice. We all became one body—a body of prayer, a true singularity.

I calmly watched us become one through all of our breaths—she came back into her body. She survived without any brain damage, which was remarkable considering how long she had been under water! Yogi Bhajan said that she had truly died and been reborn, and that the day was her new birthday. That day I understood what my father meant by feeling calm in the face of death. Most people doubt the possibility of miracles, like the Red Sea parting or the leper being healed. I don't. I have personally experienced the laws of nature altering. From that brief moment in time, I know the profound power of the word and the depth of devotion and prayer.

All of these examples are testament to the realization that there is more going on than our physical senses typically experience. People go to great lengths to have that transcendental experience. But all too often, the wrong path is taken to gain it—for example, the use of psychedelic drugs gives us a glimpse of this reality, but at the expense of our minds, bodies, and nervous systems. One of the consequences of the hippie movement was that too many people had opened their Third Eye while living in unhealthy body-minds.

They became spaced out, keeping them from their true destinies. One could say that the Guru brought Yogi Bhajan to America to heal the Woodstock Nation with the power of Kundalini Yoga.

Although it is possible to gain consciousness quickly, sustaining it requires constant fortitude. Maintaining a welcome home for your personal Guru requires daily renewal. I do my sadhana, which covers me for that day. I don't have to be perfect; I only need to act correctly enough, and the Guru covers the rest. I constantly listen for guidance; but first the chakras must be awakened and cleaned so I listen to the Guru's guidance. I recite *Japji (Song of the Soul)* daily. When I speak the words of Guru Nanak, my listening grows deeper. When I relate to Guru Gobind Singh, I gain the courage to act on the Guru's wisdom. In Yogi Bhajan's poem "Heal Me," he says, "Love, live, and be alive, ten bodies, seven chakras, three Gunas, and Tattva's five."[38] The components required for the success of the kundalini's awakening are in this poem. The subtle and the gross must be balanced, and the energy must be awakened. Expand into the light, receive the drop of nectar from His kindness, and become the God-human.

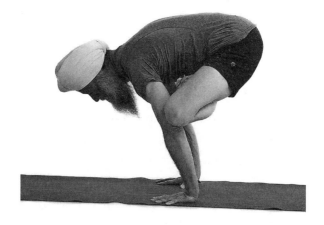

38 "Heal Me" a poem by Yogi Bhajan which Guru Prem put to music at Yogi Bhajan's request. Nirinjan Kaur is the vocalist; it's one of the 14 songs on the Therapy Series available from Invincible Music.

Chapter Six

Love: The Fruit of Kundalini Awakening

With so much that has been said about love, what more can I add? It's a feeling, it's an act, it's an emotion; but in our culture, it's primarily a commodity. Love sells. From pop music to cars to Valentine's Day candy and cards, love is everywhere. Then there's the love found in religion and spiritually: the love of God for us and our love for God, along with love thy neighbor. And in romantic love, we fall in and out of love all the time, or so we think. But love also exists in and of itself. It needs no context or application; it simply is. Love exists without our help. Love is a power.

Let me start by dispelling some common misconceptions regarding love. We don't create love, make love, or fall in love. We participate in love. Love is the way we experience truth; love is the way we experience God. Truth is that which never changes. Love never changes but we can change in our participation. When we act in love, we add to the beauty of our lives.

When we learn to do things with love, we merge with that love. The wisdom to "obey, serve, love, and excel" gives us the formula; and like any formula, we can repeat it. We can experience the science of the form and learn how to obtain the form of love and its virtues. The power of love releases us from the prison of fear. Love can make us true, kind, brave, warm, lighthearted, and so on. As we act, so we become. We obey with devotion; we serve the world; and we love all forms as the manifestations of God's love. The better we become, the easier it gets. With love of the discipline, we excel and begin to move toward ease, which flows from love as we grow in wisdom and expertise.

It has been my experience in a relationship, we don't actually love the other person; we love our own fulfillment. Most people think they are in love if they have a comfortable, though dualistic, relationship with another person. This love often means simply enjoying the feeling of being with or thinking about another person. It's true that just thinking about someone can create the feeling we call love. But feelings change. In fact, love can change to resentment, anger, and even hate because what we call love is based on duality. Most relationships are based in this love, which differs greatly from a love that is the fruit of commitment. This love, born of commitment, takes on the form given by the Guru, continually expanding and growing in the infinite and limitless identity of the formless creator, God.

What I am describing is a marriage. This marriage is based on the trinity of two bodies and one soul, all living in the grace of the Guru's guidance. The goal of the spiritual marriage is to become two bodies and one soul. As we learn to live for another human, as a husband or wife, we reshape our consciousness. Marriage is really the yoga of family life, the *grist* ashram. The Gurbani word *grist* has the same root as the English word *grist*, as in mill. Marriage grinds and refines the ego so that we can live in the infinite flow of life and love, merged in one another.

The Guru says: "They are not husband and wife who only sit together. They are called husband and wife who have one light in two bodies."[39]

Marriage is also a metaphor for our relationship to the Guru. More specifically, we are all brides longing for our husband, the Infinite God. In this way, the *Siri Guru Granth Sahib* models the kind of love we can experience in the world and in our relationships, which is through service. Through the grace of the Guru and the gratitude that it imbues in the heart, we serve humanity selflessly and, in this way, come to know true love. We can only experience love when we become capable of sacrifice. The word *sacrifice* means "to make sacred." When we offer our bodies, our time, and our energy as a sacrifice, when we love selflessly, we are fulfilled, and this fulfillment is the gift of love.

Remember that *Guru* is defined as "the One who moves us from darkness to light." With the Guru's guidance, we can synergize relationships and bring light to the heart of those who participate with us in love, merge with us in love, and, by our sides, know fulfillment because of love.

39 Siri Guru Granth Sahib, page 788, Guru Amar Das

Seven Steps to Happiness

Yogi Bhajan taught that happiness is a seven-step process that *begins* with commitment. If you love someone, you are committed to that love, and that commitment builds your character. If the relationship is based in something formless, changeless, and thus immortal, then your character will take on those same qualities. You become *akaal moorat*, or deathless personified. Your love becomes timeless, and your relationship lives eternally—the quixotic and much sought after endless love.

The three gifts of character are dignity, divinity, and grace. People of dignity recognize their own value and love themselves because of it. How they share their value is their dignity. We have various expressions about dignity: "He brings dignity to the office of the president." Or, "I won't dignify that with an answer." Self-love is dignity personified, while divinity is the power that transcends personality. Love of the transcendent moves us toward our divine nature, where we experience our grace. When we are graceful, we move smoothly and with ease. We experience the sense of being covered, taken care of, protected. Our actions and words are connected. We experience our own integrity. Grace allows us to recognize God's formless immortal nature among the myriad forms. With grace we have the power to sacrifice, by doing, living and being sacred, happiness is acheived.

To explore the qualities of grace more fully, I like to think of it as an acronym:

G is for grounded: to root and receive the energies necessary to grow. This quality represents love's sacrifice. A seed offers its self to be transformed and expand downward to receive the Earth's blessings.

R is for Relax: to relax is possibly the highest form of wisdom. Turning off the unnecessary tensions so you can feel the hand of God guiding you, relax your thinking so you can hear God's words of love for you—this is *sunni-ai,* when we deeply listen and hear the lover's voice, the whisper. Knowing and experiencing God's love, we are able to surrender what no longer serves us and, with patience, receive what is destined for us.

A is for align: to align with the Guru's wisdom and to experience the love of God's name. We are aligned when we realize and experience that God's name is not a mundane, earthly sound, but a wave, a vibration of divine love flowing from truth. This alignment allows the polarities of earth and heaven to deliver us to our true home in the heart. From this seat, we receive the treasures of God's love, which allows us to embrace the limitless resources that follow.

C is for connect and commune: to connect and commune with the creation through our creativity. From the comfortable seat, or *asana,* of the true heart, we contribute to the beauty of God's creation. I love it when I'm asked, "How do you do that?" Whether gymnastics, yoga, music, or any skill I have, I get to create community and connection just by sharing what I love. I feel the presence of God's love when I share. In fact, the greatest antidepressant for me is to share my soul through my gifts, talents, and energies.

E is for Ease: to live in *sahej* and enjoy the flow of God's infinite love. To truly be at ease in my being, my walk, my interactions, to trust in the flow of God is my greatest asset as an ambassador of the Guru's grace. To enjoy means to be with joy. My smile is my projection of joy and the summation of my experience of God's love. My presence heals. My projection uplifts. I live and let live.

This is grace.

"And They Lived Happily Ever After . . ."

Marriage is the most challenging of all "yogas." Here are some tools for success that I've discovered over the 20 years of my "happily ever after" marriage.

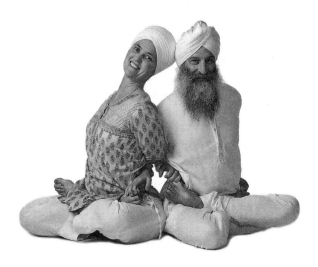

I've always enjoyed living in a comfortable environment—that is, when I am home, I wish to live a simple, cozy, and well cared for life. I prefer not to have to do too much with regard to basic household chores—cleaning, laundry, repairs, gardening, or other tasks around the house. Don't get me wrong, I appreciate them; I like to use my time at home to enjoy my family and develop myself; and I've had great success for the most part. The house is clean and cozy, and I am very blessed to be able to put my time into other things. It should be noted that this is not achieved by an overworking partner, but rather by my wife's ability to gracefully cover these jobs or to get the help she needs. My marriage, which is based in spirit, has been fun, satisfying, and happy. However, at first, I had a great deal of spiritual training to do as a single person. If you are not successful at being single, then you'll have a hard time succeeding at being a couple. By first becoming the soul-bride of God, you learn to relate intimately to the soul of another human being. The relationship with God and Guru teaches you how to successfully relate to your own soul and ultimately the soul of another.

A man must be working on healing himself from his past neuroses if he wishes to avoid major conflict in his marriage. Marriage will continue the process; but if the basics haven't been achieved, the relationship will suffer. Man represents the water element. The water element fills in the form of the feminine, the earth. My wife carries my true form within her. About 22 years ago, Yogi Bhajan interviewed me, asking what I wanted in a wife. I recall going through my list of qualities of this and that, and then he stopped me and said rather pointedly, "What you need is a wife you can lose yourself in." Lose myself? Up to that point, all of my relationships had been so neurotic that all I had lost were my time, money, reputation, and nearly my faith! A common mistake in the relationship between a man and a woman is that the woman loses herself in the man. This often results in a harmful imbalance, sometimes resulting in a dysfunctional patriarchal household.

The word "man" is contained in the word "woman". But for the man to lose himself in the woman he must do three things: be the spiritual leader of the family; provide for the security of the family—that is, provide the necessary resources and protect the family with his life; and be able to put smiles on the faces of his family. In our path, we have a saying: "Happy wife, happy life." These three principals have served me in living a healthy, happy, holy life, and they can serve you, too. But keep in mind—I'm only addressing the man's role. Writing from the woman's perspective would require a different author, and a much larger book.

I am the spiritual leader of my family. What does that mean, and why is it so important? I live the virtues of the heart. I'm true, kind, warm, brave, pure, and so on. I directly and consciously connect to the source of my virtue, my soul, every day. This is my foundation. I have a daily practice that keeps me connected to the source of my virtues and creates a constant flow of life and love in all my actions. Every morning, in the hours before the sun rises, that quiet time when one can deeply listen, I practice prayer, meditation, and yoga. I put God and Guru first in my day. I proclaim our family's identity by my own actions. My wife knows that my devotions define me, and she carries that definition with her grace and through her own practice. My wife recognizes this devotion to my true self, my higher consciousness, and thus I gain her respect. What she may not be aware of is how much I struggle in maintaining this practice! But doing it is enough, because acting good is halfway to being good, which is why it is a practice, and not a perfect.

A man without the means to provide for his family pays a price. It will eventually cost him his own comfort. A man must learn how to develop his talents and skills to serve both his family and the world beyond. When his skills are valued and he's paid well for them, his esteem rises, and his positive projection creates a prosperous green energy in his aura, providing for his family's needs and more. Part of providing is protecting. Even though my wife has years of martial arts training, making her a far better fighter than I, I still create the effect of a shield by my presence. A man can at least project the intention that he will sacrifice himself for the safety and good of his family, even if circumstances never demand it.

A man must know how to put a smile on the faces of his family. If you have been doing the first two, these skills will develop naturally. My kids smile when I come home. Sometimes it's enough to be seen and hugged; sometimes it means spending some one-on-one time with them. The warmth of your presence can be felt by listening and giving advice or just playing around and dancing. By being devoted to your own true self, you can serve with devotion the true interests of your family. You may still need to be the bottom line on occasion, but your family must never doubt the warm heart underneath.

In the end, the dynamic between husband and wife is simple: A good woman loves reflecting a good man. Men, in turn, want their partners to look good because their wives are a reflection of them. So, to enjoy longevity together and continue to grow in each other's company, both socially and intimately, it's important to maintain physical vitality. The practice of yoga and meditation strengthens both the body and the mind, which are necessary to sustain years of smiles. Yogi Bhajan said, "Women want a sexual saint". . . . "And any man who cannot satisfy his woman is a nuisance to himself."[40]

A man of virtue earns the privilege of losing himself in his wife. With yogic vitality, patience, and skill, he can bring a special smile to his partner. The yoga of this physical union, when graced by a conscious commitment, brings a smile of fulfillment like no other. Spiritual discipline not only develops your potency but also makes your virtues have more impact. Sex is a sixth sense; a function of the pituitary. Therefore, prayer, meditation, service, and yoga make a man truly potent. From these, he fulfills his oneness, and his family, in turn, feels fulfilled.

Sikh Dharma has taught me to be the sun in my family's life—that is, to be physically, mentally, emotionally, and spiritually stable. Kundalini Yoga has given me the vitality and radiance to fulfill that role with grace and ease. On this path, I am becoming bright, warm, and constant. This is true love.

40 Bhajan, Yogi. (2008) Man to Man. Santa Cruz, NM: Kundalini Research Institute.

Chapter Seven

The Power of the Word

In the beginning there was the Word, the Word was with God, and the Word was God.

—John 1:1

The most powerful and beautiful thing about being human is our word. We receive more blessings and curses based on what and how we speak than anything else we might do. Yogi Bhajan said, "Your thinking is based on what you normally speak. If you speak the word of God, your thinking pattern will become Divine."[41] The word is vibratory; it's the sound we use to communicate our thoughts, feelings, and intentions. The word *communicate* has its roots in the word *commune*. When we speak, we commune with ourselves and

41 Yogi Bhajan Everyday calendar, Nov 20, 2010; from source dated July 10, 1975

others. Effective communication builds community—not only the community within our mind, body, and soul, but also the collective community of the world around us. We are always communicating, either with our written or spoken words or silently through body language, facial expressions, and even our thoughts.

What brings power to words? Consider a typical profane word. The same word in another culture may have no negative meanings or connotations. The F and S words in English began as a sound, and vibration became empowered as we associated the sound with the power to degrade or humiliate. Like most teenagers, I used profanities with regularity. That was part of my overall speaking and unconscious exhalation processes. I was quite unaware of what came out of my mouth. Soon after beginning Kundalini Yoga, however, I made a point not to swear, unless the situation warranted it. Sometimes so-called bad words have healing powers. When I was younger, my parents did not allow me to swear in front of them, but for one exception: If I injured myself, swearing was permissible for a brief period, such as right after stubbing my toe. On those occasions, it felt good to swear. Even today, I find that a carefully used profanity, at the right moment can be an effective aid in moving the energy of a conversation. Profanities carry the power of the collective belief that they are bad; thus these special words have more power then we are usually aware.

The same holds true regarding the names of God as given by the Guru. Guru Nanak empowered Sat Nam, changing it from a pleasant sound to a divine delivery to God. The vibration of Sat Nam already vibrates at the heart, but without the empowerment of the Guru, Sat Nam is limited to being just a soothing sound. I believe that as a community holds the faith and devotion to the divine names, the power of the name increases.

As our form changes, so does our vibration and communication. Our consciousness is expressed through our form; the human body is our instrument. All the characteristics of a musical instrument, an orchestra even, live in the human body. The secret is to know how to play the music through tone, body language, and word choice. When we speak, we contract in order to shape the breath and make the sounds. These sounds can be sacred or profane, and they expand and contract accordingly. Thus, we must remain conscious of the vibrations that form us, the sounds that surround us and resound within us. Because we are always changing, how do we influence those changes for the better? We do so by listening to and speaking those vibrations that serve our soul.

We must learn to vibrate our heart's virtues, our heart's deepest truth. If we can listen to and act on the subtle voice of the soul, true transformation can occur. Before the soul can effectively transform our minds and bodies, however, we must reform our behavior. We need to purify the pathway that lies between our soul's truth and the mind and body's experience; we require "reform" school.

When I was child, my parents would occasionally threaten to send me to reform school if I didn't change my behavior. I doubt they were ever serious, but the strategy—invoking fear—worked to get me to improve my behavior. Yet, this taught me to be good by repressing bad instead of healing it. My real "reform" school began with the study of Kundalini Yoga. That was when I began my journey of healing the "bad" and transforming the mind-body-soul connection. It was where I learned to properly move, breathe, stand, sing, and speak; I began to behave in a more conscious fashion.

Our breath mechanizes our emotions, reflecting our feelings and giving them form. Being short-tempered often leads to shorter, shallower breath patterns; while patience and security are reflected in a long, deep, smoother breath pattern. As the breath solidifies emotions into form, this form is projected, further influencing and communicating who we are and how we feel. In the past, I would express myself without considering the effects or the outcome of my words. On one hand, I was honest; on the other hand, speaking honestly without subtlety presents its own problems. How you feel about something or someone today can change tomorrow. When you put your feelings into words, the communication cannot be retrieved. If you speak and hurt someone over a temporary burst of agitation or anger, the damage may be irreparable. Feelings change, so we must be careful about putting our feelings into words.

As my transformation continued, I found other tools to improve my communication. One tool I use daily is the way I dress, which communicates the person I wish to be. My Soldier-Saint uniform informs the world of my commitment to live sacredly. The way I dress also influences how I speak. My words must match my appearance. *Bana*, the way I dress and present myself, is the template I use to remind me that my commitments require sacrifice.

Consciousness Is Caught

By speaking consciously, we can clear a path to success and fulfill our destinies, whereas unconscious speaking leads to failure. We are constantly vibrating, and this vibration cannot be stopped, though it can be influenced, for better or worse. It is important to remember that we have no power to start or stop vibrating—that is God's alone. We can influence the tempo, pitch, and harmonics. We can speak the same words with kindness or cruelty. In fact, whether we use humor or anger can give the same words completely different meanings. Yet the power that brings sound to life is not ours. This is explained in Guru Nanak's *Japji Sahib*. The line, *Akana Jor Chupe na Jor*, which means, "No power to speak or silence to keep," speaks to this fundamental lack of power. Yet we do have the choice to define, refine, leverage, and guide the vibration into a communication that moves us and others toward our destiny or our fate.

Humans imitate members of their families, neighbors, and cultures. The way we speak and the accents we develop reflect the environments in which we live. I believe the only universal language is calmness, which means that when the speed of the inhale equals the speed of the exhale, that is calm. Yet there is always some emotion to our words; there is always some feeling in our speech. But when we sit and calmly breathe, emotions return to neutral. Anything else is based on opinion or experience. Our culture also influences our emotions and inflections. But calm is always calm. That is why there is no such thing as Beverly Hills calm, or for that matter German calm, but there is such a thing as Italian anger, two Italians arguing are recongizable by just their body language. The language we speak and the words we use influence our form. That is how culture informs and conforms us.

We usually speak on an exhale, and in that way, the exhale comes to define our lives. With skill we refine our intentions on the exhale. Words are the most powerful tool we have to define who we are and where we're going. So, too, our posture sets its form on the exhale. An effective breath requires that the thoracic diaphragm move freely. The heart rests just above this diaphragm, so every word we speak vibrates the heart. The way we speak, breathe, and move the diaphragm can stress or strengthen the heart. When the exhale isn't engaged correctly, it can cause the diaphragm to collapse downward, along with the heart and the weakening posture that follows. Learning to align the spine so that our speech is empowered by the pelvis, navel, diaphragm, and throat allows us to support the heart physically, emotionally, and spiritually. I have said it before, but it bears repeating: *How* you hold your heart is very much influenced by *what you hold in your heart.*

"If you remember that God sits on the tip of the tongue, you will be very watchful what you are going to do with it. The tongue is not a small thing, it lives in the thirty-two teeth. It is the most flexible part of the body, the most sensitive, and the most effective part of the body. A word said by the tongue can cut through the heart, which no medicine can cure. And sweetness from this tongue can bring you the total wealth of the world. That is the story of cause and effect, of the vibration and what it can do."[42]

I experience an embrace of my heart and soul through the exhale. How we speak and how we exhale either clears the darkness or adds new shadows to the Heart Center. On the inhale, we either expand and embrace the world with love or we might brace against the world because of our own shadows. True self-love lies in the Guru's words. When we can embrace the grace of the Guru, we are guided back toward the true word, in which we merge. As a Sikh, I live by the guidance of my Guru. In fact, it is not possible to be a Sikh without a Guru. My Guru is the *Siri Guru Granth Sahib*, which was born of the song of man.

When we speak we must learn to speak from our navel our original self, as Yogi Bhajan said. Most people have an exhale that disconnects them from their Heart Center. Few people use the navel to help ascend the diaphragm properly towards the heart while exhaling. In Latin exhale is *expiro*, or expire. This word also means death, which occurs when we breathe out our last. Yogi Bhajan commented, "You lose all happiness in life because of

---

42 Oriental Beauty Secrets, A Thought for the Day Cards by Yogi Bhajan, "Power of the Word"

the fear of death. A person in fear and phobia has no intuitive sensitivity."[43] Our fear of death affects the exhale, which, in turn, affects communication by subconsciously weakening the exhale. Although exhaling can be a conscious form of dying, it is a death to the limited ego and an awakening of the deathless soul.

Speaking from the Navel Point supports the heart, reduces the commotion and duality in our speech, and creates harmony. When Yogi Bhajan used the word *commotion*, he spoke to the reality of emotions moving in two different directions, often in conflict and disharmony with one another. Commotion and disharmony produce friction, stress, inflammation, disease, and reactive behavior, while using our communication to produce harmony adds to the beauty of the world. When we speak from the Navel Point, we can more easily speak to the Heart Center and create understanding. Yogi Bhajan often broke down words to get to their root; for example, to understand means that we must learn to stand under. When we speak truly, we stand under the true heart and speak, carry, nurture, and promote the truth by "standing under" it. Thus, we must learn to carry the true heart on a *palanquin* of devotion and vitality.

One way that we elevate our spirits through the word is when we sing it. In praise, our voices ring out, and our song becomes a resounding offering to God. In return, His gift to us is the breath, the divine inspiration. Words of truth lift the shadows of doubt. Songs of God's praise dispel our fears, which brings us to have faith in the words of the True Guru. Doubt is a disease; the Guru's words heal that disease—that "distance from the ease." Singing the words of the Guru offers a path to our exalted selves. The exhaled breath brings with it fearlessness, while the inspiration gives us the energy to experience and transcend our feelings and emotions, to

43 Yogi Bhajan Everyday calendar, November 16, 2010; from source dated, March 12, 1989

rise above the trance. As fear leaves, courage comes. Having the capacity to act with courage is fundamental to becoming a realized human being. Yet we often act and speak from insecurity, which creates new cycles of cause and effect. For example, if the exhale carries with it our sadness and insecurity, the inhale gives energy to that feeling, and we begin to act sad and insecure. If the exhale is full of fear, the inhaled breath reflects that fear, increasing it and bringing energy to it. When we lose spirit, we experience despair. When we breathe shallowly, we contribute to this lack of spirit. Joyfully praying, singing, and serving in the company of the holy keeps us from despair. Thus, the inhale and the exhale are the first movers in the law of karma—that is, we get what we put out.

Finding My Voice

Singing has always been one of my greatest challenges. For many years, it was physically uncomfortable for me. My navel only knew how to support my head, and my throat suffered because of it. I emotionally held on to so much from my past. My emotions often fought with my consciousness, creating restrictions in my face and my throat. For much of my early life, I suffered ear, nose, and throat problems. I know now that these problems were related to my issues with guilt and shame. Before I began a life of regular devotional singing, I used to feel insecure about singing, especially in public because it made me feel so exposed. I felt every weakness, every lie, every insecurity. I felt that all my defects, all my karmas, were on display when I sang.

Some years ago, I took voice lessons. Those lessons were my first exposure to my voice as a reflection of my emotional past. Part of my sound came from my parents and other close relationships. To this inheritance, I added my own ego, personality, and neuroses.

This confluence of background and individuality became my sound, and it often got stuck in my throat. I felt exposed when I sang on my own. But in the company of the devoted, I became comfortable singing. I learned to sing and chant as one voice with the congregation. Singing in the congregation of the holy can heal neuroses in our communication. Singing the words of Nanak in the company of the holy, we become Nanak. When we recite *Japji Sahib*, we become Guru Nanak, because Guru Nanak recited it. Because the Guru presides in wisdom, we bring forth the voice of our souls and sit and sing in the Guru's presence. There is no middleman. Instead, we bow to the word, and we are blessed by the word. To be blessed by the Guru's word is to become the form of the Guru. This is how, with God's grace, we will re-form the world. Aligning with the True Guru, our words and actions are refined and defined by the word. The Guru says, "Your command is upon my head, and I no longer question it."[44] The head is guided to bow to the heart; the intellect is moved to serve the heart's wisdom; and the body becomes home to God's word, no longer a slave to self-will.

How do we move from the Guru's word to our own communication? How do we embody the wisdom, patience, and tolerance of the Guru's grace? We need to be educated in how to communicate. Without intuitive sensitivity, we are clueless. How can we retrain our speech and body language? Kundalini Yoga offers many techniques to develop our communication skills and become conscious in our communication. Conscious communication demands more from us. It's not just our responsibility to communicate clearly; we must also take responsibility for the other person's understanding. It is the responsibility of the conscious person to make him- or herself

---

44 Siri Guru Granth Sahib, page 338, Line 14, Saint Kabir, 15th Century Sufi Saint

be understood; it is not the responsibility of the less conscious person to understand.

Years before the existence of the internet, Yogi Bhajan said that we would suffer from information overload. Too much information would limit our ability to recognize truth, and our words would soon lose their context and, with it, their meaning. Too much information can deform us. For the soul to be transformed, we need to be reformed in the image of the Guru. Life flows in the karma of sequence and consequence. Living the word of the True Guru, living in dharma, we can break the cycle of karma and merge with the true word. This is grace.

The Nature of Truth

In physics, *truth* is defined as "that which never changes." But what in the physical world never changes? What we see as solid and immovable actually moves and decays over time. For example, within a large rock, atoms are quickly changing, even though we don't see it with the natural eye. The dance of the atoms is very dynamic; the trinity of the neutron, electron, and proton are moving constantly; and the forces exerted from the outside change it, too. After many years, the rock becomes unrecognizable.

Until recently, it was believed that the only constant, the only truth, in the scientific world was the speed of light. Albert Einstein's quantum theory of $E = mc^2$ requires the speed of light to be constant. New discoveries, however, are indicting that the speed of light may not be as constant as once believed. The universe is a mystery of forms both subtle and gross, known and unknown. Because those forms change, they can't, by definition, be true. So what is wrong with our definition? What really is true?

Yogi Bhajan was a pragmatist, he understood that truth was in relationship to the world around it. It was in relation to the perspective of the individual, the group, and the universal. So truth causes change, and yet it's changeless. There is an old saying from India: "The secret to health and wealth is circulation because that which does not move stinks." Our bodies' various systems must circulate to remain healthy and vital; that which does not circulate decays. Here is the puzzle that must be solved in order to move forward: Truth is that which never changes; but if truth does not move or change, then truth must stink! How do we resolve this? All things are born of truth, but the truth is not born. Truth is outside of space and time, it is not created therefore cannot change, decay or die.

The great mystery of creation is how forms of life were born from the formless. Can all the vast and lively creation really come from nothing? Admittedly, this defies the laws of physics, but not the laws of God. Learning to live as Nirankar—the form of the formless, the immortal identity—is our path. We can represent ourselves as deathless personified, *akaal moorat*. Even the words we speak come from the formless. When we speak the unspoken speech, also known as *naad*, we hear the unstruck sound, the *anahat*, the immortal sound deep within the heart, resonating without beginning or end. The longing for this experience brings us to the practice of Kundalini Yoga, which cultivates within our sensory self a thrill of the subtle and a dependence on intuition.

Can something formless exist? If so, how do we recognize it? If reality requires form and nothing more to exist, then there is no truth. If truth doesn't exist, then the pursuit of virtue is just a temporary ego trip, something to make us feel better before we die. If that is the case, then our motto would be, "It's only wrong if you get caught." There would be no ultimate consequences for anything. So there must be something guiding our lives that is higher than truth. But what could be higher than truth? The Guru says, "Truth is higher than anything, but truthful living is higher still."[45] We long to live and act from our authenticity, our True Heart. But to succeed, we must be guided by the True Guru.

Thus, the path of righteousness only begins with truth. By planting the formless seed of truth into the fertile domain of the human heart, with all its light and all its shadows, even our painful and sometimes ugly pasts become valuable. We can grow a destiny from the compost heap of our past actions and plant the seed of Sat Nam, making truth our identity. The name of the formless truth, Sat Nam, is the sound of the true heart. To be human is to become the form of the formless. The true heart gives birth to the hearts of virtue. With the True Guru's guidance, we experience truth by living truthfully. We become kindhearted, warmhearted, brave-hearted, and all the other virtues. We offer it all, even our ego, to the Guru. By grace, we are accepted and we become One.

The journey to the pure heart originates in a deep longing to belong. We want to belong to something, anything. We distract ourselves with romance and social position, even religion. But what we really long for is already within us; we long to belong to that which is nearest and dearest—our own soul. But somehow we have trouble getting there on our own, even though it's within us. This is the great paradox. We can't recognize what's already our own, so we rely on its reflection outside us. We look for a form of God that we can meditate on, imagine, and love. This is the Guru.

45 Siri Guru Granth Sahib, page 62, Line 11, Guru Nanak Dev Ji

Aspiration to Prosperity—A'spira' to Pro'spira'

Our power lies in our longing. We often resist this power within ourselves because it's often a source of pain, a reminder of our loneliness. But whether it is longing for *maya* or a longing for truth, this longing is nevertheless a source of motivation; a mover in our lives.

This longing is also known as aspiration or *aspira* and is defined as what the heart and the spirit long for. Our power to attract depends on whether we have the clarity of purpose to bring into our lives those things we want, a better life not necessarily a bigger life. In a world where most of us feel overwhelmed and lost, it's easy to lose ourselves, forget what we truly want, or never identify it in the first place. Our longing attracts things; it's the power that moves things toward or away from us. There's an old saying, "Be careful what you pray for; you might just get it." We can long to accomplish things, we can long to obtain things, but the longing must be in balance with our destiny. The Guru awakens us to our soul's purpose, guides us toward that balance, and offers the equanimity of the peaceful heart. Without the Guru's guidance, we would spend a great deal of time longing for things that have limited or temporary value, which causes shadows and impurities to develop.

What I wish to share is the Guru's formula for prosperity, for a prosperous spirit. Guru Amar Das, in the *Bani, Anand Sahib* said, "God is my capital; my mind is the merchant."[46] A prayer of prosperity emanates from your own true heart to the Soul of creation. If you follow these steps correctly, you will pro-spira, or prosper.

Let's begin with the root word for this formula: *spira*, or spirit. This is the pure spirit of God—in essence, the formless creator. God's

46 Siri Guru Granth Sahib, page 921, line 8, Guru Amar Das

spirit takes form from the respira (respiration), or the respiratory system, of the whole universe. The shared great breath is in all of God's creation; it is also the human breath of life. The great respira connects us all in oneness. This connection circulates atoms and molecules of everything. We have little bits of the good and the bad of all who are here now and all who came before. Although these bits are small, they can become all, because "all is in the small." The Guru gives clear guidance for our prosperous expansion. The Guru guides God's resources to the good in you. Without the Guru, our misguided emotions could attract resources to the bad.

When our heart's longing finds success, *aspira* becomes *prospira*—that is, we prosper. Our greatest prosperity is to become truly human, the light of the mind, being. Then our spirit flows and grows. To better understand this concept, we must begin by recognizing our relationship to our own power. As an ego, we command 20 percent of our own power—10 percent is given to the other person, and the remaining 70 percent is the Great Respira, or Holy Spirit. Our individual power moves only through the Great Respira. We are connected to what we long for through the breath. Once the longing plants its vibration in the heart, it draws to us what we long for.

Begin this exercise by asking your heart what it truly desires—in other words, what is your aspiration, or *aspira*? Plant the seed of your desire by doing something good, like making a charitable donation or doing a service. You must learn to give in order receive. You must also learn to receive the feelings of your heartfelt desire in order to bring life to your aspiration. Doing so will, in itself, give you the feelings of heartfelt prosperity. As the heart vibrates these feelings, you will begin to attract what you aspire—thinking rich is not as powerful as feeling rich.

Once the feelings are heartfelt, your words and presence will carry the vibration to the world and beyond. And the beyond responds by sending conspiras. Our heart's longing draws other spirits, known as *conspiras*. *Conspiracy* is a neutral term, literally meaning "with other spirits." These other spirits—human or more subtle—come to help manifest what your heart longs for.

The gift to you transpires—comes from spirit *transpira*—from the conspiracy, or *conspira*. Are you capable of receiving the gift that God wants to transpire to you? Or are you too full from the past with lust, greed, anger, pride or attachment? If you are too full of the past, then there is no room for the "present," or gift. So empty yourself through the *expira*, or exhale, with God's name on your lips. To expire means death, and death needs to come to your past so there is room for the present and the future destiny it brings.

The gift transpires to the emptied you. As breath enters as inspiration, or *inspira*, you have the inspiration to achieve your heart's longings. You have what you need. You receive the present, and the gift is in you. But then what? True inspiration feeding your heart's desire will surely manifest prosperity if you do one more thing—you must sweat, preferably with a smile. That is the perspiration, or *perspira*. You must do the discipline as a service to your true self. Earn righteously by the sweat of your brow and share. The only thing you have to be vigilant about is guarding your spirit from despair, or *dis-spira*. Don't become dispirited and break your heart's connection to your spirit. Remember that God is your capital, and Guru is the banker. Guru lets you know how you can spend God's resources. With that understanding, your mind can be the merchant.

We give the word, the truth, a seat in our hearts, where the Guru finds a comfortable seat and makes a home. The Master of Hearts embodies the light of God and the templates of all the virtues. These virtues are the embodiment of the Guru. We speak, sing, dress, act and serve as the Guru. Our individual conscience merges with the Guru, and we join the Guru in the comfortable seat, the throne of consciousness, our own heart. We become one with God. We make the right effort, we put one foot in front of the other, and we turn the "Big Wheel" of karma. Through perspire, the sweat of our brow, we invite *prospira*. We balance effort with flow and live by a kind of quiet grace, a subtlety that arises from intuition and the self-sensory body.

Prosperity Meditation[47]

Kundalini Yoga as taught by Yogi Bhajan®

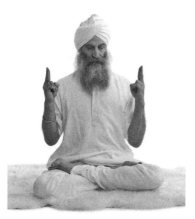

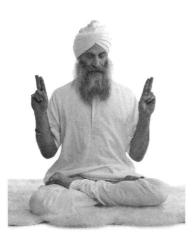

Tune in with Ong Namo Guru Dev Namo. Sit comfortably with a straight spine in easy pose or in a chair with your feet flat on the ground. Extend the Jupiter (index) finger and Saturn (middle) finger together, fold the thumb over the ring and pinkie fingers. Bring your hands up and tuck the elbows by the ribcage, the palms are facing away from the body. Chant *Har* and rotate the hands 90 degrees so the palms face each other. Chant *Har* and turn the hands so they face away from the body again.

47 © 1992 The Teachings of Yogi Bhajan

Keep repeating this motion, chanting *Har with each movement.* To maintain the rhythm, you can use *Tantric Har* by Simran Kaur.

The eyes are nine-tenths closed and focused on the tip of the nose. Continue in a steady rhythm for 11 minutes.

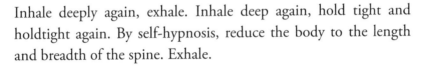

To End: Inhale deeply, hold tight, and squeeze yourself. Consolidate yourself—*pratyahar*—become zero—*shuniya*—under all circumstances.

Imagine you are just a central line and the two sides of your body have squeezed into the central line for the length and breadth of the spine only. Exhale.

Inhale deeply again, exhale. Inhale deep again, hold tight and holdtight again. By self-hypnosis, reduce the body to the length and breadth of the spine. Exhale.

Inhale deeply again, hold tight. Self-hypnosis is a very powerful thing. Exhale.

Inhale deeply and release the breath. Inhale deeply and release.

Finally, inhale deeply to full strength and hold tight as if you are just one stick that is two and one-half inches wide and the length of your spine. Exhale and relax.

Giving of What You Have

An example of faith is in sharing what I earn. A fundamental creed of being a Sikh is to earn by the sweat of your brow and to share. I have learned to give about 10 percent of what I earn to different charitable causes, because 10 percent of what I earn belongs to the Guru. But learning to let go of money was a big part of my growth.

I believed that the purpose for my early college education was to prepare myself to earn enough money to do what I wished so I could have what I wanted. I only gave to charities out of guilt. Tithing 10 percent seemed painfully impossible when I first began to give, because I had fallen into the *prosperity* trap. I believed that I would become generous when I became more prosperous. In other words, "I'll give when I'm rich." But I have since learned that the very word prosperity translates to "pro spirit." If your spirit flows, things flow to you in greater abundance. Coveting abundance before you give will ultimately deny yourself true fulfillment. In fact, it is possible to have wealth and no prosperity. If your money is growing and you are shrinking, then you're wealthy but not prosperous.

The most important thing I've learned about giving is that I am not giving my own money. Charitable giving is the Guru's money; I'm merely returning it. In a way, I help operate the Guru's bank account. Before we can expand into prosperity, we must contract. A law of the universe states that contractions create expansion. A conscious and intelligent contraction allows us to predict the expansion. In today's world, money has become a verb, meaning it's essentially backed by faith in what it does, and not what it is. Our one dollar bill says, "In God we trust." So money is what it does. When we invest it somewhere, we hope that it will help a company expand their profits, and the stock will prosper. The same is true when I recite the Guru's words: I must contract to make a sound. This contraction creates an expansion of the Guru's presence. When I let the Guru's words go from my mouth, my ego is taken from me and the distance between God and me is lessened. Thus, the contraction allows us to let things go—in this case, letting go of money that is really the Guru's money so we can receive greater abundance.

Let me describe a few events that helped heal my spirit and move me toward true "pro-spira," or prosperity. I knew I needed the faith and courage to let go of my money fears in order to become truly generous. I slowly learned to listen to where to give. I enjoyed listening to some Christian broadcasts, even though I never considered myself a Christian. One day in 1980, I was listening to a radio broadcast of a slightly eccentric but charismatic Christian preacher named Dr. Gene Scott, who was preaching on the need to show faith in giving. He said our experience of God was limited by our fear of giving. He challenged his listeners to test their faith by sending money to his ministry. I thought to myself, "He's right! My fear of giving is keeping me from truly experiencing God." So I decided right then to send Dr. Scott 50 dollars that I didn't really have. Strange that although I was living as a Sikh, I made my first act of courageous giving to a church I had little interest in. But the reason I gave there instead of my local community was that I wanted to test a pure act of faith. I gave simply because I heard someone sincerely asking.

At that time, I was working in a warehouse, doing shipping and receiving. After donating money—money that I didn't really have to give—to that Christian ministry, I felt the strength to ask my boss for a raise. This job was part of a Los Angeles Sikh community business, and I was earning three dollars an hour. I wanted a fifty cent raise, because I thought I was being vastly underpaid for being a college graduate.

But when I asked for a raise, I was turned down. So I decided to quit! Being unemployed was not what I had expected to be a result of my first act of courageous giving. But it didn't last long. I had already begun a part-time massage therapy practice. The week that I quit the warehouse job, the man who had been so instrumental in my somatic therapy career, Dr. Soram Khalsa, called to ask if I could help him with his injured back. I said sure. After my treatments, he quickly got better. From that point on to this day, he has kept me busy, sending clients who need my services. Ever since I have continued to develop my capacity to give from my heart and wallet. Giving to the Guru in God's name is the most sacred contraction guaranteed to expand your bank account and your spirit.

Chapter Eight

The Four Cornerstones
of a Great Life

On this path, the four cornerstones of a great life are known as *seva, simran, bana,* and *bani*—service, remembrance, projection, and wisdom. In order to change our life from fate to destiny, we must act consciously and selflessly.

Seva

Destiny requires sacred action, which often means an act of service to the Guru. This act of service is known as *seva*. Service is made sacred because it requires no return; the only reward is in the act itself. Learning how to serve, learning how to do *seva*, begins as just that—a conscious act. Put simply, show up somewhere and lend a hand.

My first experience of *seva* was in 1977, when I was training to be a drug rehabilitation counselor in Tucson, Arizona. Part of the program involved running a free kitchen that served the needs of the poor and indigent. Five days a week, food was prepared by the staff and the recovering addicts. We served it freely with a smile, and nothing was asked in return. It was there that I learned how to prepare food with a smile on my face and a song in my heart; the service became a meditation. In *seva*, you lose yourself in the love of the service, and the self you lose becomes part of a bigger self, which you merge with and belong to forever. Thus, *seva* leads one to become selfless in the service.

In my experience, the *seva* of selflessly serving food is possibly the fastest way to change our lives. This simple gesture begins to open our hearts and transform us in ways that are difficult to anticipate. To look in the eyes of another human being and gracefully serve him or her food can rewire the soul's connection to the mind and body. When we mindfully prepare the food, when we put our prayers into each chop of the blade, each stir of the pot, each knead of the bread, we merge our Self into the food, which then merges with the people. We create a connection, and any sense of separation drops away. We become selfless but also Self-less; we are given the opportunity to experience and sense our oneness with all living beings by being a part of this most basic human experience—nourishing ourselves and one another.

Seva is also a great antidepressant. To lift another's spirit is to lift your own. The *seva* that we render to God and Guru begins to remove the dark shadows from our hearts and reveal our own inner light. When we practice *seva*, we put our hearts in our hands, and the hands that serve the Master of the Heart also serve humanity. As our sense of posture improves, we experience the alignment of a supported heart and the hands that serve. We embody the Guru's word and become the body of the Guru by doing his *seva*. We render service to the Guru by doing his service. In many ways, *seva* is the easiest meditation. As the head bows to the service, we begin to merge into the meditative state of *sahej*, the easy acceptance of the Guru's work and God's will.

My deeper relationship to *seva* began as an obligation to the community where I live. I would show up to do langar preparation by helping to serve and clean up. But I did this work without truly feeling the love of being in the Guru's service. My service was rendered from my head, not my heart. It was akin to karma yoga rather than true *seva*. I would apply *tapas*, or heat, to a good cause; so some of my karma was burned off just by fulfilling my commitment. However, my motivation wasn't devotion; rather, it was a desire to maintain my status in the community. Doing good for the sake of one's ego earns one only a small "seat" of honor. (This seat of honor is also the comfortable seat of the True Heart.) So although my ego-based *seva* became part of my yoga, it never really flowered into devotion; when ego acts as the doer, the act is not fully accepted by the true heart. Still, I kept up. I was blessed by doing this *seva* in the presence of other, wiser hearts whose light infected my own darkness. I benefited from their experience, their devotion, and their humility; consciousness is contagious. As I matured in my experience of *seva*, I began showing up, humbly, with my heart in my hands, to serve my Guru.

Later, I was blessed to learn and experience true *seva* by participating in *ishnaan*, the marble washing of Guru Ram Das Ashram that takes place every Sunday morning. I began this *seva* as an obligation—yet another karma yoga. Every six weeks, I showed up at the ashram at 4 a.m. for about two hours of cleaning. As part of the ishnaan, everything must be taken out—the furnishings, the carpets, everything. Then, with the ashram empty, the marble floors are washed with milk and water. When I approached this *seva* as a duty, I did not enjoy it. All I could think about were the things I disliked about it: It was cold that early in the morning, and the floors were washed with cold water and milk. I would get wet, or worse, slip and fall on the wet marble. Another of my hesitations was the fear of reinjuring a chronically injured shoulder. A combination of old injuries from gymnastics, new irritations from my yoga practice, plus all the emotional trauma stored in my upper body made me reticent to lift those heavy carpets. But the worst part was that everyone else seemed to really enjoy doing the *seva*. Why did I feel so differently? I began to think that those who "en-joyed" must be serving with joy. They were not eccentric; the problem was within me. My attitude and approach to *seva* were penance, payback for my past sins and karmas. I was there to suffer, and my ego felt the need to make a good show of it by doing *seva*.

In my life, I have been blessed with many miracles. But *ishnaan seva* blessed me with several. When I realized the problem was within me, I decided to do an experiment: I would go each Sunday for six straight weeks to find out if I could change my attitude or at least find the source of other participants' joy. During those six weeks, improvements began to appear. I started to enjoy being there, and to my surprise, my injuries began to improve. This small miracle kept me coming back, and I started to learn the basics of *seva*— how to be in the presence of my higher self and serve. A simple act of offering my body and mind to clean a house of the holy offered the profound gift of witnessing the Guru's presence through that same simple act. I chanted God's holy name and served the house of the Guru. And my reward? I witnessed God's presence through the Guru within my own body, and I learned to serve those who come to bow at the feet of the Guru.

Simran

Simran, the second of the four cornerstones of a great life, means to meditate on the names of God (Nam Simran). But what does it mean to meditate on the names of God? The constant repetition of a sound, which represents the divine qualities of God, draws his attention to our consciousness. We become soul brides to God by taking his Name to heart. God is fully conscious of us all, but we are not fully conscious of God. Nam Simran allows us to call upon God's name, which opens us up. It's as though we are knocking on God's door, and we keep knocking in the hopes that God will begin to hear us. We believe that if we just keep knocking, the gate of God will one day open. But it is really the other way around. If we keep knocking, one day we'll open. This "knocking" occurs when we bow our heads and repeat God's holy name with every breath. As we open up, we learn to listen through the deep listening known as *sunni-ai*. As we quiet our noisy minds, we can leave our thinking behind and listen with our hearts.

Simran is also the act of planting the name of God in the "soil" of the true heart. But what does this mean? Metaphorically, the Guru instructs us on how to prepare the soil of our body-mind to receive God's name. Any skilled farmer will tell you that the soil is more important than the seed. If we just repeat God's name without skill and devotion, then very little will grow. The Guru instructs the ego to behave divinely in order to receive the name and to merge in the consciousness we call God. So we knock on the door of God until our hearts open, then we plant the seed of the name and grow in *akaal purkh*, or deathlessness personified.

Knowing the science of Nam Simran makes the experience far more effective, which is why proper alignment and technique within the practice of asana and pranayama are so important. Kundalini Yoga combines all of these elements to achieve the skill necessary for successful Nam Simran. Yogi Bhajan always reminded his students to chant from the Navel Point. To be able to properly access the Navel Point, however, we must first know how to sit comfortably with a straight spine. The Navel Point empowers the breath, which creates the resounding effect of Nam Simran within the body, helping to define and refine the heart's virtues. These technical aspects allow the seeker to leverage devotion and empower action, meditation, and *simran.*

As mentioned earlier, our actions influence the way we think, feel, and behave. We project this form to the world, and the world responds in kind. Life looks like us. When done properly, *simran* allows us to leave the prison of our dark hearts and emerge from the shadows that distance us from our own destinies. We created those destinies, and we can change them through one act of surrender, one act of devotion. Nam Simran opens our heart to God's light, and the shadow lifts from this one act of grace.

Another essential result of Nam Simran is the transformation of the heart and its renewed longing for a personal guru. When we open up our hearts through divine chanting, we expand in relationship to gravity. We take on new forms, and the Guru provides the *template* that defines that new form. As explained earlier, the word template translates as "the form of the temple." If the body is the temple of God, then the Guru has given us the template to make that body, that form, into an image of God that we can "meditate on, imagine, and love."[48] The Guru gives shape to the divine virtues, and we, in turn, take God's Name to heart and embody the virtues as the form of the Guru.

---

48 Japji by Guru Nanak English Translation by Guruka Singh Khalsa.

Meditation for Anger and to Wipe Out Mental Negativity [49]

Kundalini Yoga as taught by Yogi Bhajan®
June 15, 1982

A meditation to help you see things clearly; without emotion.

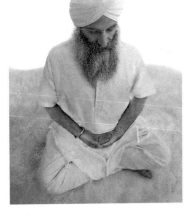

Posture: Tune in with Ong Namo Guru Dev Namo. Sit in easy pose with a straight spine. Relax the hands in the lap, palms face up with the right hand resting in the left. Touch the thumb tips together.

Eyes: Closed

Mantra: *Whaa-hay Guroo, Whaa-hay Guroo, Whaa-hay Guroo, Whaa-hay Jeeo.* Inhale very deeply. As you exhale, chant the mantra 8 times per breath, in a monotone. Breathe very deeply in order to complete the cycle, which will take approximately 45 seconds. Release the breath very slowly as you chant. Each syllable of the mantra must be pronounced very distinctly. You have to say it a little fast to be able to repeat 8 times on one breath. If at first the breath doesn't hold for the full 8 repetitions, stop, breathe and begin again. Build up your capacity.

(continued on next page)

49 Kundalini Research Institute (2009). The "Last Resort" Meditation in I Am a Woman: Essential Kriyas for Women in the Aquarian Age. Santa Cruz, NM: KRI, page 110.

Time: This meditation can be done for 11 minutes for the first few days, then increase to 22 minutes, and gradually build up to 33 minutes. The day you can spend 2-1/2 hours chanting this mantra in a monotone, you will be a totally different person. Nothing can defeat you then. You will accomplish your goals on the spiritual path, and all weaknesses will be gone.

Comments: Practice of this kriya will enable you to think right, act right, see right, look at yourself, imagine, meditate. Everything else follows. You will wipe out a lot of negativity.

When done in the cycle of eight times per breath for 11 minutes, this meditation will build in you courage, commitment, and strength.

When life doesn't work for you and you don't want to go to anybody, practice this meditation. The mantra means, "You are Beloved of my soul, Oh God." It causes a very subtle rub against the center of the palate. It stimulates the 32nd meridian, known in the West as the Christ Meridian, and in the East as the Sattvica Buddha Bindu.

Meditating with this mantra can help you to understand the meaning of a yogi. When you perfect the state of consciousness, it will start giving you the joy of drinking honey. The taste and the feeling of honey comes in your mouth, in your body, and in your whole system. You feel very sweet. That is when you know it has started working. It is not only the pituitary that starts secreting, but also the pineal gland. There is also a little arc called the "moon of the brain," and there is a little membrane filled with juice. That is the juice you usually carry to death. That turns and you drink it. Death doesn't bother you and you don't bother it.

The tenth Sikh Guru, Guru Gobind Singh, did this meditation for eleven months and eleven days near Anandpur.

Guru Prem's Comments: Breath of Fire for a few minutes before you begin can help you to successfully do it. What I have always enjoyed about this meditation is that it pulls you out of your head and into you heart. It does this by overpowering your thinking. In other words, it empties your head. Do this meditation when you are very stressed and can't seem to get out of your head.

Bana

The third cornerstone of a great life is *bana*, or identifying ourselves as beings of consciousness. With the Guru's guidance, we "act as if," we "walk the walk," we live according to the form of the Guru within us. For me this entails a formal standard of dress, which helps to identify myself in the public world as a being of consciousness; I try to dress in a way that reflects that standard of consciousness. Each path has its own standards, and everyone expresses that standard in his or her own way. But imagine if you looked into the mirror each morning and consciously decided to dress for God—not for your family or a date or a business colleague.

Do we dress to impress, or do we dress to create an impact? The idea behind *bana* is to compliment and reinforce those elements that deliver us to our own souls, amplifying the light of the soul by the choices we make and how we represent ourselves to the world. We can dress in a way that *complements* our consciousness rather than *compromising* it.

There is an age-old question of whether the clothes make the man or the man makes the clothes. I believe it can be both. How I am as a man, how I stand, and what I stand for all influence what I wear. For me, the body beneath the *bana* is just as important.

How I care for myself—my mind, body, and spirit—contributes as much or more to my radiance as the *bana* I wear. *Bana* serves as my public interface with the world. To live in the world as a householder requires being with people of every consciousness. In a world where the heart's shadow is often greater than its light, innocence needs to be protected. But how do we know who can be trusted and depended upon? My outer form and inner strength serve and protect those who cannot protect themselves.

> The bana was given by the Tenth Sikh Guru; it is the template of the Soldier Saint—a soldier's body and a saint's heart. By standing out in a conscious manner through the bana, I am telling the world to hold me to a high standard. The world and its myriad forms bring to bear a certain pressure, sometimes more intensely than others, which test my commitment to the excellence I represent. If I choose to stand out, then I need the support of a strong body and mind to withstand the outer pressure and come to balance. Kundalini Yoga does just that. Flexibility, strength, and steady nerves are required to live in the world as a conscious human being. The real underpinning of bana is to be as good as you look. Make yourself beautiful before God, and by Guru's grace, become as good as you look.

Living to this high standard is a big part of my "off the Mat or sheepskin" meditation. People of character must know what they stand for; in fact, their commitment to standards is what makes up their character. In turn, their commitment to character gives them dignity, divinity, and grace. Knowing that they dwell in the grace of God grants them the privilege to sacrifice. This sacrifice, this sacred act, opens the heart to happiness. So, for me, *bana* is the ultimate symbol of my willingness to sacrifice.

The practice of Kundalini Yoga molds and tempers me to conform to this *bana* and to feel the presence of the Guru within the discipline of it. So, too, my physical strength is the Guru's strength. My flexibility allows me to stand straight and create space for the Guru's presence. I dress for that presence—the presence of the Guru within me. All who truly believe that God dwells in their hearts have an obligation to represent that presence to the world. Our dress, posture, and language define our presence. How we care for and love ourselves greatly influence how the world cares for and perceives us.

I am neither a fanatic, nor am I lazy. I simply allow myself to dress appropriately for the occasion. But mostly I dress for consciousness. This doesn't mean that I always dress formally, because I don't. Every activity has a conscious standard. I don't wear *bana* when I ski; so when I ski, I don't stand out in any special way. But my manners and my kindness, my posture and projection speak for me. Many of you may be asking, "If you behave so well, then why do you need the clothes to tell your story?" Well, this particular form tells the world that I am available; I'm ready to be of service, and the light of my virtues is more easily recognized. Because my ski clothes don't enhance my projection, I have to be more aware of my behavior.

Dressing consciously didn't begin when I put on Guru Gobind Singh's *bana*. When I think back on my development, I see a series of uniforms that greatly influenced my young life. When I was about seven years old, I studied piano with a Russian teacher named Mr. Hillsberg. He was quite strict, and I was required to wear a dress shirt and tie when taking a piano lesson. I had a great fear of and respect for Mr. Hillsberg. I was afraid not to come prepared to take my lesson, so I practiced. But what I didn't understand at the time was the requirement to dress consciously for my lesson.

Putting a tie on didn't in itself make me a better musician. But learning to dress in the consciousness of being in the presence of my teacher definitely made me a better student.

At about the same time, I was a catcher on a little league baseball team. My team was the Yankees, and I loved our uniforms. They weren't professional quality, but they were good enough to make me feel that I was part of something special. That was my first experience with being part of a team. The uniform made us all feel the "oneness" of our form. This oneness of form helped create team spirit. Individual boys with some baseball skills came together to become something greater then the sum of our parts.

When I turned eight years old, I joined the Cub Scouts. The uniform had a military feel to it. I used to enjoy putting on my father's oversized military uniform, so having my own was a thrill and a real sense of pride. Wednesday's were my favorite days, because it was den meeting day, which meant I could wear my uniform to school. At my elementary school, it was common to see kids wearing Cub Scout, Brownie, Girl Scout, and Camp Fire Girl uniforms. There was pride both in the uniform itself and what we got to put on it. I worked diligently to earn my merit badges and loved having them on display on my scout uniform. I made it a point to earn all the badges—the tiger cub, bear, wolf, not to mention all the arrow badges.

After Cub Scouts, I became a boy scout. I was very excited to begin a new series of challenges to possibly become an Eagle Scout. Strangely, though, about six months into my Boy Scout "career," I became very self-conscious of the uniform. I was nearly 12 years old, and the Vietnam War was at its height. I felt embarrassed to be seen in a uniform. For the first time in my life, I felt uncool. So I quit the Boy Scouts. By then, I was already into regular gymnastic practice, so I had other activities and other uniforms. Although my gymnastics uniform was not militaristic, it still identified me as being part of a team.

During high school, I had to endure being different, because to be on the gymnastics team required maintaining a very short haircut. All of my non-gymnastic friends had long hair, but I couldn't. Even though it was very uncool to have hair as short as the team required, I survived and even thrived by being different. It's funny that for the past 34 years, I have been different because I don't cut my hair, and I am still wearing a uniform.

Would a policeman know less about law enforcement in casual clothes? No, but the projection of authority is greatly enhanced by the policeman's uniform. *Uniform* means "one form." A uniform makes the sum greater than the parts, which is why group consciousness is facilitated by wearing uniforms. The way I express myself as a Sikh is in a white uniform, and I choose to wear white most of the time, because it amplifies my impact. The color white expands my presence, projects what is good within me, and protects me from what is harmful outside of me. White contains the full color spectrum and can amplify our virtuous qualities. White can also filter out the heart's shadows, limiting their dark projection into the world. Yogi Bhajan taught that white *bana* was the most difficult thing to wear because it makes us stand out. But standing out is, in itself, a mindful meditation.

The journey from the ego's need to impress to the soul's purpose to impact has been a difficult but necessary path for me. I am learning to feed on my ego—eat it up, so that it doesn't eat me. There is always a danger of craving old feelings, even in the presence of new insight. Sometimes we use our new energies to feed old neuroses. This is the challenge of the devotee on the path of dharma. *Bana* holds me to the form of my Guru, and thus I am reminded that God is in me and close to my heart. *Bana* helps me transform my formless soul into the form of the Guru.

I don't want to conform to outside forces. Beauty can be bewitching or elevating. The outer symmetry that represents the classical beauty must be equalized by inner virtue; otherwise, ugly consequences will follow. It is a curse to be born beautiful and act ugly. If you are privileged to possess beauty in your life, then let that beauty become the standard of your excellence. And remember, how you care for and love yourself will determine how the world will care for and love you.

Bani

"Bani is not to be understood by the head; it has to be understood by the heart." [50]

—*Yogi Bhajan*

"In the beginning was the Word." The first line of John's testament in the Bible states that we came into form through the word. "From one vibration, the world came to be," this is *Ek Ong Kar*. All forms are made up of vibrations. The Guru's form is made of the purest vibration. In that state of divine oneness, we can speak the unspoken speech. Guru Amar Das talks about this in the *Anand Sahib*, or *The Song of Bliss*. When the heart is pure, we speak the unspoken. This is bani, the word of God. With devotion and a little technique, I, too, can speak the words of those who have truly been in the state of God-consciousness.

We learn and are transformed by the Guru's *bani* through deep listening, or *sunni-ai*. We learn to hear the voice of God by singing the Guru's hymns. The act of *sunni-ai* brings us to surrender,

50 © The Teachings of Yogi Bhajan, July 16, 1982

relaxation, and ease. This ease, or *sahej*, merges us into the oneness of *shuniya*, or emptiness. From this starting point—from zero—we listen and receive. From this deep listening we're able to serve with devotion and dedication, letting go of duty and obligation. We serve the Guru that rules our true heart; and with love, devotion, and surrender we merge with our Guru. Raj Yoga becomes our consciousness.

Japji Pauris: Sunni-ai

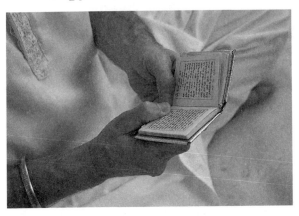

Sunni-ai sidh pir sur nath, Sunni-ai dhart dhaval akas, Sunni-ai deep loa patal, Sunni-ai poeh na sakai kaal, Nanak bhagata sada vigas, Sunni-ai dukh pap ka naas

Sunni-ai isar brama ind, Sunni-ai mukh salahan mand, Sunni-ai jog jugat tan bhayd, Sunni-ai shast simrat vayd, Nanak bhagata sada vigas, Sunni-ai dukh pap ka naas

Sunni-ai sat santokh gian, sunni-ai athsath ka ishnan, sunni-ai par par paveh maan, sunni-ai lagai sahej dhiyan, Nanak bhagata sada vigas, Sunni-ai dukh pap ka naas

Sunni-ai sara guna kay gaah, sunni-ai shaykh pir pathishah, sunni-ai andhay paveh raho, sunni-ai hath hovai asgaaho, Nanak bhagata sada vigas, sunni-ai dukh pap ka naas

> *Listening, Saints, heroes, masters,*
> *Listening, the earth, the power, the ethers,*
> *Listening, high and low realms, oceans of light,*
> *Listening, beyond time,*
> *Oh, Nanak, God's lovers bloom forever*
> *Listening destroys all pain and error.*
>
> *Listening, Men become Gods,*
> *Listening, praise comes from the mouth of the most negative person,*
> *Listening, the way of Yoga and the body's secrets,*
> *Listening, all holy books and scriptures,*
> *Oh, Nanak, God's lovers bloom forever,*
> *Listening destroys all pain and error.*
>
> *Listening, truth, patience and wisdom,*
> *Listening, bathing at all holy places,*
> *Listening, reading and reading gains honor,*
> *Listening, concentration comes easy,*
> *Oh, Nanak, God's lovers bloom forever,*
> *Listening destroys all pain and error.*
>
> *Listening, deep oceans of grace,*
> *Listening, Kings, Emperors, Saints,*
> *Listening, blind ones find the path,*
> *Listening, the unknown is known,*
> *Oh, Nanak, God's lovers bloom forever,*
> *Listening destroys all pain and error.*[51]

There is no such thing as original wisdom. Wisdom doesn't have an origin other than truth. Words of true wisdom are timeless and immortal. The true heart listens and speaks the unspoken speech. When we recite or sing the words of the True Guru, we become the vessel of the True Guru. The true wisdom of the Guru manifests as the Guru's *bani*. As we sing these *banis*, they merge head and heart, duty and devotion, knowledge and wisdom. The Guru's *bani*

---

51 Japji Pauris 8, 9, 10, 11 by Guru Nanak, translation Guruka Singh Khalsa

teaches us how to think by giving us a perfect template of divine knowledge. Because of its poetic form and the rhythm in which it's sung, we can take this knowledge to heart. Nam Simran delivers us to deep listening; *bani* develops our thinking, giving us the skill to use the positive and negative minds wisely and with neutrality.

I believe that the face is a mirror of the mind and the eyes are a window to the soul. The technology of Gurbani is used to recite the Guru's words, which we do with the tongue inside the mouth. The words alter the shape of the face to bring forth the presence of the Guru. We can't exactly imitate the sound of Guru Nanak, but we don't need to. Guru Nanak gave us the tools to help bring forth his *bani*. By singing the *bani* in specific rhythms and scales, we can come closer to the mind of the Guru. This is the science of Naad Yoga, in which the sound current can flow through our being. This devotional singing done in the *naad, sound current* of the Guru brings us into a state of *cherdi kala*, or rising spirit.

The face of God's light emanates from our smiles to elevate humanity. The truly radiant face shows the mind of God. We don't push the Guru's word on the world. We don't proselytize the Guru's word. Instead, we share the "gospel" with our smiles. The light of God manifests in the heart as the recognizable virtues. God's light sparkles out of our eyes as we "see the world through the Guru's eyes." Singing the knowledge of the Guru through his word in a congregation of other devoted people leverages the group energy to the oneness that is God. We sing as one and become one. As the old saying goes, "God respects you when you work and loves you when you sing."

Chapter Nine

The Throne of Raj Yoga: On Building a Personal Practice

Patanjali, the great yogic sage, defined *asana* as a "comfortable seat" where the soul is experienced in the heart lotus. The whole point of asana is to build, with the Guru's guidance, a comfortable seat of virtues where the Guru can sit and rule. Devotion to the One who occupies the comfortable seat brings comfort and joy. The Guru who sits in the heart lotus is the one I serve with mind and soul, breath and bone. By listening, I realized that the real purpose of my yogic adventure was to learn the techniques and take the wisdom of each asana to heart. With an open heart, we receive the gifts of the various asanas. I don't need to reincarnate as a rock to gain the wisdom of steadiness, patience, strength, and stillness. Doing *vajrasana*, or Rock Pose, with the right heart and spirit, I can receive these qualities.

I try to do everything as an offering to the One who sits on the throne of Raj Yoga. For me Sikh Dharma, the Khalsa, Kundalini Yoga, and all the other yogic supplements and complements are an offering to the Guru who rules from the heart lotus of Raj Yoga. Extending my life through yogic practices is ultimately pointless if not done as an offering to the True Guru. Twenty minutes after I'm dead, my body will be very stiff, unable to do anything. There is no honor in asanas or kriyas by themselves; they are a means to an end. The asanas and kriyas contain knowledge, and we must be humbly trained to guide the physical and other wisdoms to the heart. A yogic head trip is just another disease of overidentifying with the physical for emotional satisfaction.

Tools of equalization and transformation are the *bandhas*, which shape the breath that serves the heart. Rendering true service to the heart with a concentrated focus, or *dhristi*, eventually connects the heart center to the eyes. We say the eyes are the window of the soul, and the soul illuminates its presence in the heart. With deep intuition, we can see the world through the Guru's eyes, which is known as *pratyahar*, in which the physical senses are withdrawn, allowing the spiritual senses to see, feel, and know truth. For the heart to see, we must learn to serve the heart with both our vitality and our intellect. As we sing in the *Song of the Khalsa*, "Give our lives to God and Guru, mind and soul, breath and bone." This giving is physical, mental, emotional, and spiritual.

The muscles that serve the heart create a maternal relationship with the heart by using the sacred pelvic core and the navel to regulate the speed and direction of the breath. These muscles are the support, similar to a mother holding a baby. They hold something so sacred and special, something that must be protected, carried, and supported. The sacred core connects to the earth for leverage and to better serve the sternum and heart center. This allows us greater ease to move, turn, stand, walk, sing, jump, punch, and become carefree. This part of the kundalini process is a form of "re-mothering." Use this sacred core to bring vitality from the lower centers to the domain of virtue, the heart center. By serving virtue, we allow the true heart to grant us more vitality. This vitality leads to improved flexibility and better leveraged movement. We become smoother, lighter, and brighter in how we move through life.

The virtuous heart, through the Guru, also has the power to unlock the hidden domains of the navel and pelvis, which allow a highly refined form of energy to serve the greater needs of our destiny. In serving the heart one can also serve the domain and home of the Guru. This home is also the home of love; so, by serving the true heart, we move closer to love. This physical love is consummated by the union of the inhale and exhale. A covenant exists in the space between the inhale and the exhale—the domain of the breath that never changes; it is true. Only the rhythm, meter, and tempo of the breath change around the changeless true heart. When we practice yoga as a moving prayer, we can begin to move with love and into love. This love brings us to witness the movement from the comfortable seat of the true heart. This is where the ease is experienced and where excellence flows from.

I have witnessed a student, who was limited to practicing only from a wheelchair, experience this ease and excellence. Thus, yogic excellence is not limited to only those of great strength and vitality. Indeed, those with great vitality sometimes become the most neurotic—I know this from personal experience. To develop a yogic body in order to attract more emotional drama is to become strong at doing wrong. However, those with less vitality but who use what they have to serve virtue are far better yogis. A great quote of Yogi Bhajan's regarding this is, "If strength and flexibility were all that mattered in becoming a yogi, then all of the saints would be in the circus"

Having said that, being healthy is important—though not all-important—to our yogic progress. What really matters is that we succeed at fulfilling our destiny—that is, to go home to God through the Guru of the true, and eventually, pure heart. Kundalini Yoga doesn't deliver us home. Instead, it prepares us to be able to go home when we are called.

Kundalini Yoga teaches us to prepare for everything but to expect nothing. This preparation is where Kundalini Yoga shines in its value. My first mantra came from my experience with the Cub Scouts, and that mantra is "Be prepared." In Kundalini Yoga, we become prepared to receive gifts and blessings, but we take nothing; so we expect nothing, yet we become fulfilled. Yogi Bhajan taught that the law of the vacuum is that there is no vacuum.

We need to be prepared for when we receive the call to come home. The best preparation is the facsimile of death. Every exhale is a kind of death, and some deaths are better then others. Facing life's stressors with better breath control provides the basic tool for stress management. In other words, stress management is breath management. Refined further, I feel I'm granted life with each inhaled Sat—my true inspiration—and I go home to my heart with the offering of Nam on the exhale. This Nam delivers me to God through my Guru. All I can offer to God is my smile and my name, Guru Prem Singh Khalsa, having lived through his name. This is the foundation of my preparation for my journey home and in this way I approach my Kundalini Yoga practice.

Our intelligence or intellect must also be trained to bow in service to the true heart. The head and intellect are the paternal domain of the body-mind. When we train the intelligence and thinking of the head to serve wisdom and to listen to the heart, the true heart has the power to grant us more intelligence and clearer thinking. Intelligence serving virtue makes us smarter. We become level headed when our head and neck root into the wise heart. The intellect becomes rooted into the wise heart, creating a level platform on which to balance the head and allowing better navigation of the interests below. This navigation is far more successful if the intellect is trained in the understanding of divine knowledge. The Guru's wisdom taken to heart develops the mind of a *Gurmukh*. This thinking is in servitude to *sunni-ai*, or divine listening. So levelheaded people think less because they listen more.

Jalandhar bandh, or Neck Lock, is usually applied with some *mulbandh*, let your chest lift, so you create the space to draw your chin inward, elongating the back of your neck. This helps develop the alignment patterns to produce a level head, while also decompressing the neck in the area of the brain stem. But the neck cannot be aligned without aligning the whole body. At best, the neck and shoulders fine-tune the alignment. I like to think of alignment with this metaphor—an anchor at the base, wings in the middle (breath moving the ribs), and a golden thread at the top. This thread gently lifts heavenward. But if the chest collapses, so does the neck, and the head becomes misaligned, weakening the body all the way down to the feet as it tries to compensate. My basic belief about alignment is as follows: Essentially the aim is to expand the body's symmetrical space and fill it full of goodness. Through the tools of breath, bandhas, and dhristi we can follow the templates of correct form and alignment in order to better serve the Master of the Hearts.

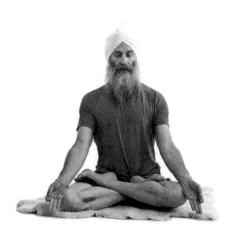

The sacred intensions of correctly doing *jalandhar bandh* open the pathways from the higher centers of the brain so they can communicate back to the heart. *Jalandhar bandh* is also important in developing the ability to correctly bow the head to its Heart Master. Using the correct techniques allows us to expand from a two-minded person to a three-minded person. My life has improved because I am better able to rule from my neutral mind with service from my positive and negative minds. The development of the three minds—positive, negative, and neutral—is exactly how we prepare for everything and expect nothing. I am still learning to act positively—and even to act negatively for positive reasons—so that I can receive grace neutrally. Praise and blame are the same to the neutral mind. To receive and experience pain without suffering is an important goal. So I practice being in pain without suffering, which can be as simple as holding the arms out parallel for 15 minutes to enjoy the pain. Be with joy and pain, but don't suffer. That is why I always try to practice with my "yoga face" on. The more it hurts, the more I smile. I love the faces of the saints and sages when they smile. I put on my Buddha face or my smiling Yogi Bhajan face or my compassionate Jesus face. That is one reason I have so many pictures and statues of smiling saints around my house. I try to copy their expressions, because these saintly faces reflect the mind of neutrality.

My neutral mind is how I receive and deepen my listening. By learning to receive good and bad neutrally, I can play the hand that I was dealt with positive and negative skills, while not becoming disconnected from the neutral. The neutral mind requires calmness, or the equalized breath. This equalization allows us to move along the path of devotion while serving our inner virtues.

Much of the physical kriyas require the ability to remain neutral while enduring discomfort. We use our positive and negative minds to pick and choose the various kriyas to explore. Then we use these two minds to safely navigate the experience. Of course it's good to maintain a posititive attitude when doing your practice. But positivity alone is not enough to become successful. For example, I might be drawn to do the You and Your Body Kriya; I'm usually attracted to something by my positive mind. This kriya begins with *Urdhva Dhanurasana*, or Wheel Pose. But starting any exercise in a deep backbend needs to be qualified by my negative mind. Am I capable of safely doing such a difficult exercise? Do I really need this kriya? These are negative mind questions that need to be asked in order to progress safely. Here are my rules for the negative mind while practicing Kundalini Yoga: Don't hurt yourself, and if you are in a class, don't let the teacher hurt you. We know ourselves better than the teacher usually does. If you don't feel safe with certain postures, then don't do them! Injuries can sometimes bring valuable lessons, but there are often better ways to learn. For most of my life, I exercised with ego; I only brought my negative and positive minds to my practices. I would do things with great positivity, ignoring the voice of caution, and I would sometimes get injured. I think my neutral mind only participated to laugh at my silliness while waiting patiently for my reconnection.

Having taken the long way to a certain degree of realization, let me share some more insights to help you progress smoothly along the way. One way to experience Kundalini Yoga is to do it on the inside, or to visualize yourself doing the kriyas or postures. I often go through kriyas mentally, because it gives me a feel for them. Just as athletes use visualization to improve their performance, you can use it to improve your meditative mind.

A great example of doing the training "inside" was demonstrated by my high school gymnastics coach, Coach Rose, who became a gymnastics coach by accident. He had been the junior football coach when he was asked to substitute for the regular gymnastics coach. He had never been a gymnast, and I doubt he ever did even a simple cartwheel. Nevertheless, he became the coach because the regular coach left. What Coach Rose learned to do was become a gymnast on the inside. He gave himself permission to do it all inside his own mind. He never physically expressed what he could do inside because he couldn't—and he didn't have to. He was quite overweight on the outside, but Olympic caliber on the inside. He was so effective with his words that we learned by the spirit of his inner knowledge and wisdom. In addition, Coach Rose would often use a student to demonstrate a skill, because he had the skill and wisdom to project his knowledge through his students, and we excelled.

I recommend approaching Kundalini Yoga in a similar manner. Learn as much as you can with your outer body and do the rest on the inside. In this way, no matter your physical capacity, whether you have an old injury or an existing limitation, you can always practice any kriya with the mind.

Examples of Kriyas I Love
Kundalini Yoga as taught by Yogi Bhajan®

Maha Padmasana

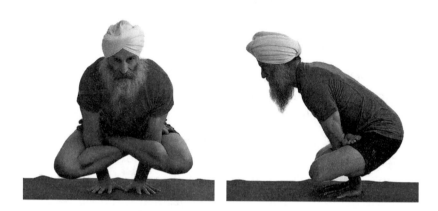

Yogi Bhajan regularly taught classes in Los Angeles. On one such occasion, Yogi Bhajan came to class carrying the April 15, 2001, edition of *Time* magazine. He began this class by talking about the cover. On the cover was fashion model Christy Turlington doing a difficult yoga asana called *kukkutasana*, or Rooster Pose. As Yogi Bhajan held up the magazine for the class to see, he talked about the power of this asana. He then renamed the asana to *maha padmasana*, or the Great Lotus. This asana requires great skill to do in full lotus, because once in lotus, you push your arms through your tightly crossed legs. The arms must extend through the lotus by about 6 inches. From there, you lift onto your hands, balance, and breathe deeply. He said to master this asana, you needed to clear the earth's magnetic field by 6 inches and stay balanced. He also said that if you mastered this posture, all the knowledge of the universe would flow into you. This is possibly the last yoga asana that Yogi Bhajan taught in his lifetime.

This is one the 84 postures that I was working on at the time, and I can tell you, it is a very difficult asana to perform correctly. As you might imagine, I was amazed and inspired by what he said about this particular asana. I could hardly wait until after class, when I might have the opportunity to ask what he meant by mastering this posture. Class ended, and as was often the case, Yogi Bhajan remained seated on the teacher's bench, talking to individual students. My wife, Simran, and I waited patiently to speak to him. When it was our turn, I asked Yogi Bhajan to explain what he meant by mastering *maha padmasana*. He leaned forward, bringing his face close to mine, and said these words with a grin and twinkle in his eye, "Do it until the pain goes away!" Then he started laughing.

So that's it—do *maha padmasana* correctly until the pain goes away. This was going to be fun! Since I could already do the posture, I just needed more fortitude, and then all the knowledge would come to me! Until then, when I had practiced the pose, I would only stay in it for about 10 seconds, because after that it became too painful to continue. And even then, I didn't have my legs the required 6 inches off the earth. But I was very determined to have an experience. During one of my practices of this asana, I used too much force while rocking into it. I came up onto my hands so fast that I knew I was about to fall over. In this posture, both hands are stuck to the ground and cannot be moved because they're locked inside the lotus posture. I realized the only thing I could do was decide which part of my head would hit the floor. I hit the side of my head so hard that I knocked myself out, and there was a moment in my unconscious state where I thought I had succeeded! I happened to be practicing yoga with a few other people who were there to revive me from what I momentarily thought was success but quickly became embarrassment. The knowledge I received was a large bump on my forehead. That experience knocked some sense into me by reteaching me a somewhat familiar lesson about not conquering the asanas. It was a lesson that I evidently still needed more practice in. Even today, I continue to practice *maha padmasana*, and it still hurts, and the knowledge is still out there.

Bowing Jaap Sahib

Tune in with the Adi Mantra: Ong Namo Guru Dev Namo. Sit on your heels and place your hands on your thighs. An acceptable variation is to place your hands on ground; in addition, there is an advanced method, done with the hands interlaced behind your back. With the hands clasped and shoulder blades drawn together, extend the arms up and lift them away from the back each time you bow forward. Regardless of the variation you choose, bow your forehead to the ground with devotion and in rhythm with the mantra.

When bowing, keep the head in alignment with the heart. Begin by slightly bowing the head to the contents of your heart, elongating the spine, coming into Jalandar Bandha, this can help prevent over flexing the thoracic spine. As you exhale, stabilize the navel and bend from the hip joint and fold forward. On the inhale, root your

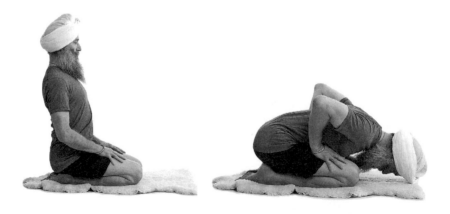

navel, knees and feet down into the ground to begin, this will help make your heart feel light and the head will follow as you come up—heart before head. When we lift the head first it compresses the neck and lower spine and you won't be able engage the power of the navel properly. If you do this exercise while chanting the same physical mechanics apply but are no longer coordinated with the breath.

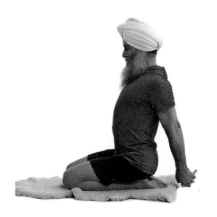

This practice is ideally done with Jaap Sahib. However, it can also be practiced while listening to the mantra, Chattra Chakkra Varti, which is the final slok of Jaap Sahib.

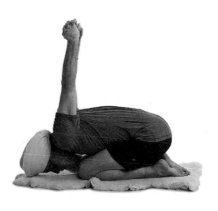

Put the music on and move to the rhythm of the sound current, you are taking the essence of the word, the Naad, to heart. Use this mantra whenever your grace, your power or your position are threatened. Start by practicing 11 mintues.

This bowing meditation can also be done to the entire Jaap Sahib meditation, which is even more powerful because it takes about 31 minutes to complete. Jaap Sahib describes the very essence and nature of God.

Gorakh's Kriya

Let's talk about how to approach Gorak's Kriya with the proper spirit and technique. I have a great personal fondness for this Kundalini Yoga Kriya. It is unique because of the way it strengthens and opens the hips and lower spine. *Gorakh*, who was believed to be the incarnation of Lord Shiva, is held in the highest regard as one of the greatest yogis. Born in the 11th or 12th century, he founded a school of yoga for devotees living the renunciate life. When Guru Nanak had his conversation with the yogis, *Siddh Gosht*,[52] they were devotees of Gorakhnath, and even today, followers of Gorakh's teachings are called Gorakhnaths. These yogis were known to have great mystical powers, called *siddhis*, which, according to Vedic wisdom, are the supernatural skills that yogis can develop.

The body usually begins to age at the sacrum. The five sacral plates become more compressed because the muscles of the pelvic floor are not being used correctly. The muscles of the pelvic floor weaken because they are not being used to connect the sit bones or the feet properly to the earth. The pelvic muscle also weakens because of emotional and sexual difficulties. In addition, the sacred domains weaken from incorrect information about the proper use of the navel-pelvis. Without this area supporting the thoracic diaphragm, basic alignment cannot be properly maintained. As the pelvic muscles weaken, so does the sacrum. Then the hips began to tighten, because they have to work harder to hold the body up against gravity. We begin to use too much peripheral tension because of an insufficient amount of properly applied, intelligent central tension. As the hips overtighten, the pelvis shifts from its correct alignment, which affects the feet, the head, and the neck. The head then shifts out of alignment. With both the hips and the head out of balance, the spine suffers. We then sit, stand, and

---

52 Siri Guru Granth Sahib, page 938-946, Guru Nanak Dev Ji

walk poorly, trying to compensate with the smaller muscles of the upper body and fighting the larger, stronger muscles of the lower body. We remain unaware until we feel pain. This is how the body generally ages—in essence, we are as old as our spine.

These misalignment patterns begin as feelings that are influenced by everything from genetics to what we ate for breakfast. Feelings move to form by the rhythm of the breath; that is the motion of emotion. Gravity then compresses our feelings to form. We start to look like we feel.

This kriya addresses the aging patterns at their beginning. Done properly, Gorakh's Kriya can help us reclaim, improve, and increase the function of the pelvic floor, hips, neck, and spine. If you have limited flexibility, proceed with caution. This is an advanced kriya.

Tune in with the Adi Mantra: Ong Namo Guru Dev Namo.

Posture:

1. Sit calmly in Celibate Pose, with your buttock between your heels. 2 minutes.

   Guru Prem's Comments: If you have difficulty with the knees, sit in vajrasan on the heels or sit on a yoga block or place a pillow between the feet under the hips.

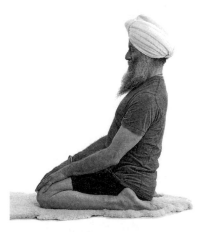

Your breathing can be improved by using the power of the *bandhas*. The *mulbandh*, or Root Lock, can help guide the inhale down to open the diaphragm muscle and pelvic floor at

(continued on next page)

the beginning of the breath. As the inhale continues, use the *uddiyana, the flying up movement,* to spread the ribs out and around into the sides and back body. The *mulbandh* continues to facilitate the expansion of the midbody along with the *uddiyana.* Applying a light *jalandhar bandh* allows the upper ribs to open as the chest lifts to the top of the inhale. Reverse the process as you exhale. While exhaling, always keep the navel point engaged to give support to the heart center. This allows the speed of the exhale to remain the same as the inhale.

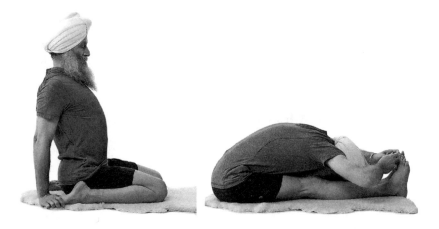

2. Stay in Celibate Pose, reach back and grab the toes. With the arms straight, begin a spinal flex. Breathe as slowly and deeply as you can and move the spine rapidly. Move the spine unsynchronized with the breath; ideally rocking the spine up to 40 times per minute. 2-3 minutes.

To End: Immediately stretch the legs out in front and bend forward at the navel without collapsing the thoracic vertebra and hold the toes. Inhale deeply, exhale completely and engage the bandhas. Hold the breath out for as long as you comfortably can. Do this only one time.

Guru Prem's Comments: The *uddiyana bandha* creates a powerful vacuum effect. The power of the fully engaged *uddiyana bandha* strengthens the internal organs by compressing them deeply, which, in turn, facilitates a basic detox by wringing out the tissues.

3. Relax for 2-3 minutes.

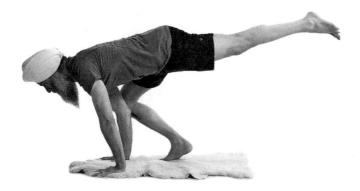

4. Begin in a squat position. Place the hands flat on the floor. Lean forward and lift the left leg up and back, parallel to the floor, with the toes pointed. Lift the chest; the weight is balanced between the two hands on the ground and the ball of the right foot is pressing down into the ground. Hold this side for 30 seconds; then change sides. Continue for 30 seconds per side for three cycles on each side.

    Guru Prem's Comments: This posture brings great heat to the hips, which will be put to great use in the asanas that follow. In this posture, it is important that you attempt to hold your chest up and one leg up and back, parallel to the ground, balancing on both hands and the ball of the foot.

(continued on next page)

5. Sit and bring the soles of the feet together. Then pick yourself up and bring the sit bones forward until they rest on your heels. Keep the soles of your feet touching while maintaining this seated position. Once your sit bones and heels are settled, bring the hands into touching position where you can be safely balanced. Meditate at the Third Eye with long deep breathing. Stay for up to 3 minutes and then relax for 2-3 minutes.

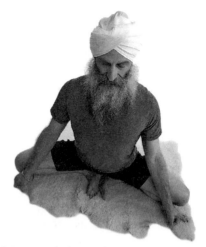

Guru Prem's Comments: This is the jewel in the crown of this kriya—*Gorakshasana*. This is a very advanced asana when done correctly. That said, there are many modifications that make it possible to experience it at its essence.

The best way to approach this asana is to put something very soft under your feet to ease the considerable pressure that will be placed on them. Then place your hands behind you and lift your hips off the floor. Begin moving forward and back as you slowly begin to move your hips to your feet.

Another method to enable the experience of *Gorakshasana* is to use a foam yoga block. Start by sitting on the block with your soles pressed together on the floor. Slowly slide off the block as you move your hips toward your heels. The power of *Gorakshasana* is a deep connection with the spirit of Gorakh. Although the posture is physically challenging, the essence of the asana is subtle. The wisdom and conscientious of Gorakh are vast.

Gorakh was much like the Buddha—calm and powerful. Many believe Gorakhnath to be a True Guru. Faith in the spirit of Gorakh while doing this asana will bring you to the deepest detachment. In addition, the asana, when done with the proper devotion, can unlock the powers that lay deeply hidden in the navel, hips, and pelvis.

6. Begin by standing with the feet 2–3 feet apart. Squat down and place the palms on the floor. While keeping the balls of the feet on the floor, pivot forward, bringing the forehead to the ground on the exhale. Then inhale up. Continue for 2–3 minutes. This will deeply open the hip and strengthen the upper body.

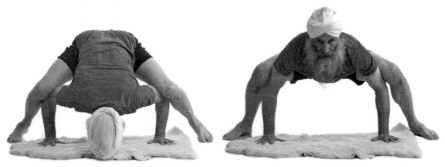

Guru Prem's Comments: This exercise is a dynamic form of *Bhekasana*, which is a form of Bowing Frogs. *Bhekasana* is a powerful example of putting devotion in the motion. Having received the blessing from Gorakh's asana, we can now take that experience and offer it as a blessing to our own souls as we bow in reverence. This asana is also a good example of moving vitality to virtue. The hips and pelvis open and move the energy to the heart. The head is also involved, as it bows in service to the heart master.

7. Sit in a comfortable meditative position and meditate on the Self—pure and transparent. Project out mentally. 3-11 minutes.

Afterword

A Personal Prayer and a Hukam from the Guru

My prayer for you dear reader is that you may find your True Guru, that you may listen deeply to your own inner voice, and that your inner wisdom may guide you to your destiny. It is my prayer that on reading this book, you were entertained, you learned something, you tried at least one of the exercises, kriyas, pranayams or meditations, your spirit was elevated and finally that you feel empowered to walk on your path of destiny.

May we all live in joy, and may we share the love that's in our hearts through the actions in our lives and the smiles on our faces.

Raamkalee, The Word of Bayni Ji

੧ਓ ਸਤਿਗੁਰ ਪ੍ਰਸਾਦਿ ॥

One Universal Creator God. By The Grace Of The True Guru:

*The energy channels of the Ida, Pingala and Shushmanaa: these three
dwell in one place.*

*This is the true place of confluence of the three sacred rivers: this is where
my mind takes its cleansing bath. ||1||*

*O Saints, the Immaculate Lord dwells there;
how rare are those who go to the Guru, and understand this.*

The all-pervading immaculate Lord is there. ||1||Pause||

What is the insignia of the Divine Lord's dwelling?

The unstruck sound current of the Shabad vibrates there.

There is no moon or sun, no air or water there.

The Gurmukh becomes aware, and knows the Teachings. ||2||

Spiritual wisdom wells up, and evil-mindedness departs;

the nucleus of the mind sky is drenched with Ambrosial Nectar.

One who knows the secret of this device,
meets the Supreme Divine Guru. ||3||

The Tenth Gate is the home of the inaccessible, infinite Supreme Lord.

Above the store is a niche, and within this niche is the commodity. ||4||

One who remains awake, never sleeps.

The three qualities and the three worlds vanish, in the state of Samaadhi.

He takes the Beej Mantra, the Seed Mantra, and keeps it in his heart.

Turning his mind away from the world, he focuses on the cosmic void of the
absolute Lord. ||5||

He remains awake, and he does not lie.

He keeps the five sensory organs under his control.

He cherishes in his consciousness the Guru's Teachings.

He dedicates his mind and body to the Lord's Love. ||6||

He considers his hands to be the leaves and branches of the tree.

He does not lose his life in the gamble.

He plugs up the source of the river of evil tendencies.

Turning away from the west, he makes the sun rise in the east.

He bears the unbearable, and the drops trickle down within;

then, he speaks with the Lord of the world. ||7||

The four-sided lamp illuminates the Tenth Gate.

The Primal Lord is at the center of the countless leaves.

He Himself abides there with all His powers.

He weaves the jewels into the pearl of the mind. ||8||

The lotus is at the forehead, and the jewels surround it.

Within it is the Immaculate Lord, the Master of the three worlds.

The Panch Shabad, the five primal sounds, resound and vibrate there in their purity.

The chauris - the fly brushes wave, and the conch shells blare like thunder.

The Gurmukh tramples the demons underfoot with his spiritual wisdom.

Bayni longs for Your Name, Lord. ||9||1||

From one vibration the world came to be,
from this mantra into eternity,
we all dance to this song of God,
let's join hands and carry it on.

Ek Ong Kar, Sat Nam, Siri Wahe Guru!

Glossary

A

Ambrosial Hours. 2 1/2 hours before sunrise.

Amrit. Nectar of Bliss.

Anahat. Unstruck sound.

Apana. Elimination, the eliminating force, cleansing breath of life.

Asana. Comfortable seat, Yogic posture.

Aura - Auric. field of subtle, luminous energy surrounding a person or object.

B

Bandh (bandha). Lock or gate.

Bhakti. Yogic path of devotion.

C

Chakras. Energy Centers.

D

Dharma. Path of Righteousness.

G

God. Generator, Organizer, and Destroyer (or Deliverer) of all Creation, God is a "word".

Gurbani. The Guru's word, language that the Siri Guru Granth Sahib is written in and meant to be sung in Raag, the power inherent in the sound current.

Gurdwara. Sikh Temple or place of worship: literally "gate of the Guru".

Guru. That which takes us from darkness to light. Teacher. In the Sikh tradition there were only ten human beings at that time who had the consciousness of "Guru". The 11th and final Guru of the Sikh's is embodied in the Siri Guru Granth Sahib which is treated as the living Guru.

I

Ida. Left Nadi, subtle energy channel: relates to left nostril, moon energy.

J

Jalandhar Bandh. Neck lock.

K

Karma. Action and reaction. the cosmic law of cause and effect.

Karma Yoga. Yoga of non-attachment, selfless service to clear karmas.

Khalsa. Pure one, a Baptized Sikh, a common last name taken by many Western Sikh's.

Kriya. Specific combination of yogic posture, hand position, breathing and mantra: literally a 'complete action'.

Kundalini. literally, 'curl of the lock of hair of the beloved' dormant energy that resides at the base of the spine until awakened thru practice or grace.

L

Liberation. The experience of your own infinity.

M

Mantra. Sound current that tunes and controls mental vibration; a syllable or combination of syllables that help focus the mind; words of power; mental vibration to the infinite mind.

Maya. Anything which can be measured; usually thought of as the 'illusion' that we mistake for reality.

Meditation. Letting God talk to you.

Mudra. Yogic hand position, literally 'seal'.

Muladhara. First, root chakra.

Mulbandh, or *Root Lock*. A contraction of the navel and perineum the pelvic floor.

N

Naad. Basic sound for all languages through all times originating in the sound current; the universal code behind human communication.

Nadis. Subtle channels for the flow of consciousness and the kundalini.

P

Patanjali. A Great Yogic Sage, Author of the oldest known yoga discourse (Sutras).

Pingala. Right Nadi, subtle energy channel: relates to right nostril; sun energy.

Prana. The energy of the essence of life, God's gift to you(that you receive with each inhalation. Breath is the primary carrier of prana).

Pranayam. Yogic breathing technique.

Prasad (prashad). Gift

Pratyahar. One of the eight limbs of yoga, it is the synchronization of the thoughts with the Infinite.

Prayer. Talking to God.

R

Raj Yoga. Royal path of yoga.

S

Sadhana. Daily spiritual effort or practice.

Shabad. Sound; sound current.

Shakti. Feminine aspect of God, God's power manifested.

Shuniya. A conscious state of zero.

Shushmana. Central Nadi, subtle energy channel along the spinal column.

Sikh. Literally a seeker of Truth; one who embraces the Sikh way of life.

Siri Guru Granth Sahib. The living Guru of the Sikhs; a volume containing the sacred words of enlightened beings who spoke or wrote them when they were in a state of union with God.

Siri Singh Sahib. Chief Religious Authority of Sikh Dharma of the Western Hemisphere Siri Singh Sahib Bhai Sahib Harbhajan Singh Khalsa Yogiji also known as the Kundalini Yoga Master and Mahan Tantric, Yogi Bhajan.

W

Wahe Guru. Wow! God is great! mantra of ecstasy expressing the indescribable magnificence of God.

Y

Yoga. Union: the science of yoking or uniting the individual consciousness with the Universal consciousness.

Yogi. One who has attained a state of yoga, a master of him/her self; person who practices the science of yoga.

Index

About the Author

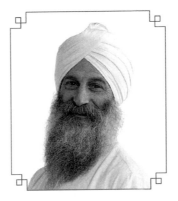

Guru Prem Singh was named Posture Master by Yogi Bhajan; he has been teaching Kundalini Yoga for more than 30 years. A Professional Trainer within the Aquarian Trainer Academy, he is an advanced Kundalini & Ashtanga Yoga practitioner and an expert in body awareness in relationship to personal growth. He travels all over the world teaching the tools and rules of divine alignment and letting your heart rule. The author of two other books, *Divine Alignment* and *The Heart Rules*, Guru Prem has had an active practice at the internationally renowned Khalsa Medical Clinic for more than 25 years, as a structural, breath, Yogic and Massage Therapist.

Guru Prem is also a musician, composer, producer and arranger, with more than 11 albums of mantra music including, *Tantric Har, Aquarian Sadhana, 'The Therapy Series'* with Nirinjan and many more! For more information see www.divinealignment.com